Simple Resistance Band for Seniors

Senior-Focused Resistance Band Training To Revitalise Health

By

Risa Denton

Copyright © 2024 Risa Denton ,

Table of Content

INTrODUCTION

I've been deeply involved in the health and fitness community for many years, and I'll be honest with you: my main reason for writing this book is a bit selfish.

I love helping people on their fitness journeys. It brings me joy to see them succeed, make positive changes in their lives, and achieve things that might have seemed impossible. Over the years, my clients have changed, but their accomplishments don't get old.

My passion lies in assisting the older population in navigating aging through exercise. Exercise is like a key that unlocks positive changes in their lives, and I believe it is the secret to a longer, healthier life. It doesn't just offer physical freedom; it also affects the social, emotional, and mental aspects of life.

I understand that aging can be challenging. The physical changes we go through can feel like uncharted territory, but I'm here to guide you through it.

Whether you're starting your exercise journey or coming back from an injury or a break, I want you to have the knowledge and confidence to face any physical health challenges with ease.

The exercises might seem simple, but don't be fooled; their simplicity is what makes them effective. You'll find a series of activities that will help you unlock your highest potential and achieve your fitness goals. They are easy to understand and simple to follow. You can do all these exercises from the comfort of your home with minimal equipment.

Before we dive in, I want to commend you for taking the initiative to regain your health and vitality, especially in a society where the narrative around getting older is often negative. We're told stories where we're supposed to lose physical and mental competence as we age, but it doesn't have to be that way. We can rewrite our stories and age with grace, strength, and independence.

I welcome the years ahead as a privilege to grow old. We become wiser, form deep relationships, and live through historical moments. We've been given full lives, and we can use the years ahead to continue living with vitality.

I understand the frustration that may come with the changes in our bodies. It can be disheartening and even scary at times. I've felt let down, scared, despondent, and angry when reaching for a jar overhead became a bit challenging, and I felt less sure on my feet.

Our bodies will go through changes—it's a fact of life. Our metabolism, bones, joints, and muscle maintenance will be affected. We might notice a decline in balance, an increase in falls, and even changes in memory and mood.

But remember, this doesn't have to be our story. We don't have to accept it. I understand it might seem challenging to maintain physical well-being in old age, and I'm confident I can show you how to navigate this chapter without stress.

Exercise can have a positive effect on all aspects of our lives—from physical and mental to emotional. It's a tool that can help you handle the challenges that come with aging. It may be challenging at first, especially as a beginner, but rebuilding your strength and improving your health is not as difficult as the alternative. All you have to do is get started, and by picking up this book, you've already begun your journey.

CHAPTER 1: GETTING STARTED

You might have seen them at the gym, the physical therapist, or your doctor's office.

What are they?

They're called resistance bands, also known as exercise bands, resistance loops, resistance tubes, or therapy bands. These stretchy bands were invented in the late 19th or early 20th century and were initially used to strengthen and expand the chest. In the mid-20th century, physical therapists started using them to help patients recover after surgeries or injuries.

Over time, athletes and fitness trainers began using them to boost strength and training. Now, anyone can buy them at various retail stores or online. In this chapter, we explore why training with resistance bands is beneficial and how it can help us. We also discuss the different types of bands available, helping you choose the right one.

Why Train with Resistance Bands?

Resistance bands are popular for workouts because they're convenient, affordable, adaptable, and easy to take with you anywhere. They're a must-have for your home gym.

These bands can be made of fabric or elastic. They work by adding tension and resistance to your movements, making exercises more challenging and making your muscles work harder. This helps build and maintain strength.

Resistance bands provide a great workout, whether you're a beginner or an advanced athlete. They are super flexible and come in various resistances, from light to heavy. Plus, they offer a safe and gentle way to exercise, providing a low-impact workout for your muscles.

Variety

You can do a wide variety of exercises using a resistance band, making it a versatile piece of equipment. Whether you're into strength training, stretching, balance, or mobility exercises, a resistance band is a valuable tool that offers excellent results.

It works almost every muscle group effectively, providing a full-body workout. These bands are great for targeting larger muscles and also help strengthen smaller supporting muscles. This leads to physical benefits like a stronger core, back, and shoulders, which in turn improve your stability and posture.

Versatility

Resistance bands are super flexible. Most exercises you can do with weights, you can also do with resistance bands. Whether it's bicep curls or good mornings, you can use resistance bands in clever ways to get a good workout. They're easy to carry around, making them perfect for travel, and they're also budget-friendly.

Provides a Full-Body Workout

A stronger resistance band is good for working your bigger muscles like the glutes and thighs, while lighter bands are great for your smaller muscles such as shoulders, upper back, and calves. You can also use them for stretching and moving around.

These bands are a bit wobbly, which makes your workout more challenging compared to using free weights like a kettlebell or dumbbell. Plus, you can do many different movements with them, giving you a full-body workout that's efficient and saves time. You're in charge of how much resistance you want, so each exercise can be adjusted to fit your fitness level perfectly.

Increases Time Under Tension

Time under tension is about how long your muscles work hard during an exercise. Take a bodyweight squat, for instance. Your leg muscles work more when lifting your body from a squat to a standing position. Now, if you use a resistance band around your shoulders and under your feet, it makes the squat tougher. The band adds resistance, making your legs work harder against it. Also, the band makes your muscles work during both the downward and upward parts of the squat, creating tension throughout the whole movement.

Burns Fat

Doing exercises with resistance, like using resistance bands, is helpful for losing fat. These exercises cause your body to burn calories even after you've finished working out. This is known as excess post-exercise oxygen consumption (EPOC), which is the energy your body uses to recover after exercise and return to its normal state.

Unlike cardio, resistance band exercises help build and keep muscle. More muscle means you burn more calories even when you're not doing anything. Muscles use a lot of calories just to stay in shape, so having more muscle boosts your metabolism, keeping it higher than if you didn't have as much muscle.

Improves Mobility

As we age, our joints, bones, cartilage, and muscles might experience some wear and tear. However, we can slow this down by staying active, moving around more during the day, and following a good exercise plan that includes stretching and balance exercises. When you use resistance bands along with your stretching routine, they can enhance the stretch and make it harder if you want more of a challenge. These bands are helpful for gradually improving your range of motion as you go through each movement and want to push yourself a bit more.

Improves Posture and Relieves Aches

Exercising helps you tune in to your body and improves your awareness of it. This awareness can lead to better posture as you pay attention to how your body moves and how you carry yourself in different situations. Understanding and enhancing your posture can also relieve some of the discomfort you might be experiencing from putting your body in less-than-ideal positions.

Reduces Risk of Injury

Resistance bands are great for beginners because they're easy to learn how to use correctly. They're gentle on your joints, providing a workout for your muscles without putting too much stress on your joints. This is especially helpful for people dealing with arthritis or joint pain.

Using resistance bands also encourages good form and proper movement. Sometimes, when people are tired, they use momentum to finish a movement or lift a weight. With a resistance band, you must rely on your strength without external help. This encourages the right and safe way to move, ensuring you only do what your body can handle.

Types of Resistance Bands

Resistance bands come in various types, with different shapes, colors, lengths, and resistance levels. Typically, thinner and skinnier bands are for smaller muscles, like the ones in your arms. They can cover more distance and move more easily. On the other hand, thicker and wider bands are for larger muscles, such as those in your legs and lower body. Overall, bands can be broadly grouped into two categories: flat or tubular.

Flat Bands

Flat bands are like flat pieces of rubber or elastic and come in different thicknesses and lengths. The flat bands include:

- **Loop bands:** These bands resemble large rubber bands and are about 40 inches in circumference. They are flat and come in different widths. The thinner the band, the less resistance it provides. For example, a band that's half an inch wide might offer resistance from five to 25 pounds. In contrast, a band that's two and a half inches wide can provide resistance from 60 to 170 pounds. These bands are excellent for full-body workouts, physical therapy, and stretching.

- **Mini bands:** These bands are the lightest, longest, and thinnest among the flat bands. They are not loops; instead, they are free bands—long strips of elastic that can be used for different exercises. Some of them can be really long, over six feet! They're commonly used in physical therapy and Pilates workouts because they provide lower resistance, typically ranging from three to 10 pounds. These bands are great for beginners with resistance bands or people recovering from injuries.

- **Therapy bands:** These bands are the lightest, longest, and thinnest among the flat bands. They are not loops; instead, they are free bands—long strips of elastic that can be used for different exercises. Some of them can be really long, over six feet! They're commonly used in physical therapy and Pilates workouts because they provide lower resistance, typically ranging from three to 10 pounds. These bands are great for beginners with resistance bands or people recovering from injuries.

Tubular Bands

These bands are like hollow tubes made of elastic or rubber, and they come in different thicknesses and lengths. These tubular bands include:

- **Figure 8 bands:** These bands have a shape like the number eight. They're tubes with a thick foam tube or ball in the middle and handles at both ends of the eight. The bands provide resistance ranging from eight to 20 pounds and are used for exercises that involve pushing and pulling. They're useful for movements like bicep curls, situps, and side lunges that involve side-to-side and forward/backward motions.

- **Tube bands with handles:** These are commonly seen in gyms and physical therapy offices. They are long elastic tubes with handles on both ends. The resistance, ranging from five to 50 pounds, depends on the thickness of the tube - thicker tubes have more resistance, and thinner ones have less. With handles on each end, these tubes can be anchored to a door or chair, offering different ways to use them. They are excellent for exercises involving pulling, like bicep curls, or pushing, such as overhead shoulder presses.

How To Create An Effective Workout Routine

To start a good workout plan, knowing your fitness level is crucial. This depends on how often you exercise, how hard you push yourself, your diet, age, and any health conditions.

If you're a beginner, aim for two to three weekly workouts, each lasting around 30 minutes. Focus on low-impact exercises with fewer repetitions and sets, using a lighter resistance band.

For intermediate fitness levels, target three to four workouts weekly, lasting 30 to 60 minutes. Increase intensity with more repetitions and sets, and use a medium-strength band.

Advanced exercisers should aim for four to six weekly workouts, lasting 40 to 90 minutes. These intense routines involve maximizing repetitions, sets, and using a strong resistance band for the highest impact.

The key to a safe and effective workout lies in proper preparation. Understand your workout goals, physical limits, and what you want to achieve. Develop a weekly routine that suits your needs. For instance, an intermediate level might focus on arms one day, legs the next, back and core on the third day, and chest and shoulders on the fourth day, with rest days in between. You can choose specific exercises but target all parts of your body equally.

Remember, rest and recovery are crucial. While exercise is about pushing yourself, knowing when to stop and allow your body to recover is equally important. Maintain a balanced diet, stay hydrated, and get enough sleep, especially after intense workouts. Create a specific time or space to stay motivated and focused for your workouts. A dedicated area adorned with motivating quotes or images of your goals can inspire you to stay consistent and use your resistance band regularly.

Repetitions

Creating an effective workout involves deciding the right number of repetitions and sets for each exercise. Repetitions are how many times you do a movement, and sets are how many times you repeat a group of repetitions. For example, if you do ten bicep curls, take a short break, and then do another ten, that's two sets.

The choice of repetitions and sets depends on your goals. For muscle strength, increase the number of sets. To focus on proper muscle alignment and activation, lower the repetitions and sets and do the exercises slowly, paying attention to your body. For endurance, increase repetitions and shorten breaks between sets.

Start with five to ten repetitions and three sets in a typical intermediate workout. Adjust based on your initial strength, endurance, or body alignment. Always prioritize safety and quality, overreaching your goals. Remember to do each exercise on both sides and ensure your workouts are well-rounded, targeting all muscle groups equally.

Quality Over Quantity

To use these exercises effectively, consider a few important tips.

Firstly, since resistance bands resist your movements, work against the band in each position. Ensure the band slightly resists your positions and movements. You can increase the resistance or switch to a stronger band if the exercises become too easy.

Focus on doing each exercise correctly and safely, especially when working out at home without professional supervision. Follow directions slowly and precisely, moving your body only as instructed. Avoid additional movements not specified in the instructions, as they can lead to injuries like strains or improper twisting.

If you move more than instructed, follow beginner suggestions and use body awareness to activate the correct muscle groups. Move within your physical limits without sacrificing form, and avoid jerking motions. Smooth movements improve muscle activation and build strength.

Pause at the height of each movement where the targeted muscle is most activated. This helps improve muscle memory and strength. However, if you experience any unusual pain, such as cramps or sharp pain, listen to your body and adjust accordingly.

When holding the band in your hands during exercises, wrap the ends around your palms and hold the excess by making fists to prevent slipping. Be cautious when wrapping the band around your body, ensuring it's not too tight, as excessive elasticity can be harmful.

Maintain a relatively tight resistance while allowing room for movement to prevent the band from snapping back. Ensure the band is securely anchored or held to avoid inconveniences like resetting exercises between sets. Holding the band too tightly or stretching it too far can lead to snapping or small tears.

Lastly, protect yourself with good-quality workout equipment, including supportive shoes for standing exercises. Supportive shoes protect your feet, which, in turn, support your back, preventing future injuries. Consider investing in a good yoga mat, especially for exercises on the floor, to provide additional cushioning between you and the hard floor, protecting your joints.

CHAPTER 2: WARM UP AND COOL DOWN

EXERCISES

Now, we'll go into more detail and share a list of warm-up and cool-down exercises that you can use to get ready for your workouts.

Warm-Up Exercises

Warm-ups have several advantages:

- They boost the flow of blood and oxygen to your joints and muscles.

- They make your blood vessels wider, helping blood circulate more smoothly.

- They make your muscles more flexible.

- They raise the temperature of your muscles.

- They activate sweat glands to prevent overheating.

- They lower the risk of injury.

- They release hormones that turn carbohydrates and fatty acids into energy.

Perform the following movements with intention and control—take your time, no need to hurry.

Start your warm-up with some cardio to get your blood flowing. Follow it up with a ballistic warm-up, which involves slow, gentle, and rhythmic movements. Choose a cardio activity you're comfortable with and pick exercises that match the type of workout you have planned.

If you're working on your upper body, focus your warm-up on that area, and do the same for your lower body if that's your focus. You can also opt for a full-body warm-up. Enjoy experimenting with your warm-up routine; there are no strict rules.

Cardio-Based Warm Up Exercises

Marching

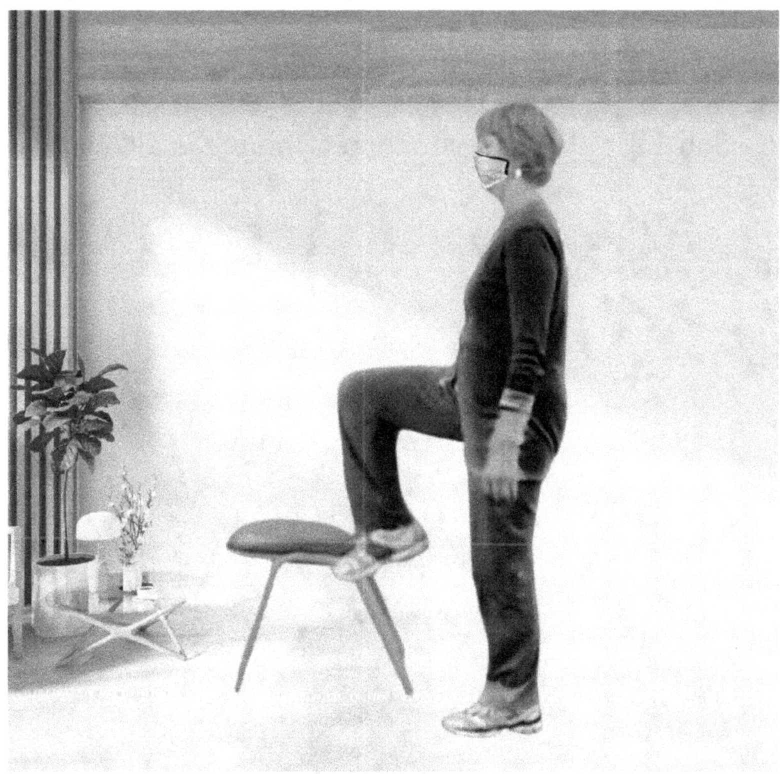

Here are the steps to do this warm up:

1. Stand tall with your shoulder blades back and down, arms at your sides, and feet under your hips.

2. Bend your knee and lift your left leg comfortably high while swinging your right arm in a marching motion.

3. Lower your left leg back to the ground and return your right arm to your side.

4. Repeat the motion on the other side.

5. Keep marching for the designated time.

6. Starting with 30 seconds to a minute is a good way to begin.

Walking Jacks

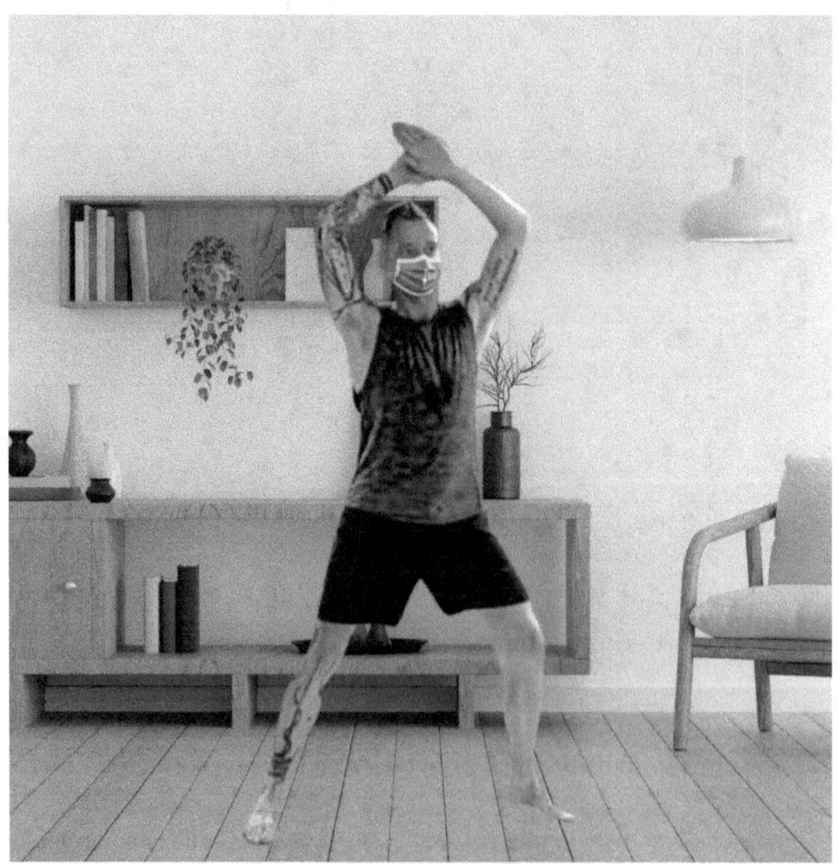

Here are the steps to do this warm up:

1. Stand tall with your shoulder blades back and down, arms at your sides, and feet under your hips.

2. Take a lateral step to the left with your left leg.

3. While stepping, swing both arms out to your sides and extend them upwards until they meet overhead.

4. Lower your arms back to the starting position as you return your left leg to the middle.

5. Repeat the motion on the right side.

6. Keep going with your walking jacks for the designated time.

7. Starting with 30 seconds to a minute is a good starting point.

Knees to Elbow Marching

Here are the steps to do this warm up:

1. Stand tall with your shoulder blades back and down, arms at your sides, and feet under your hips.

2. Bend your left knee and raise your leg as high as comfortable.

3. Lower your left leg back to the ground.

4. Repeat the motion on the right side.

5. Continue this marching motion for 10 repetitions.

6. Now, involve your arms. As you raise your leg, bring your opposite elbow to meet your opposite knee.

7. Return to the starting position and repeat on the other side.

8. Keep going for the designated time.

Shadow Boxing

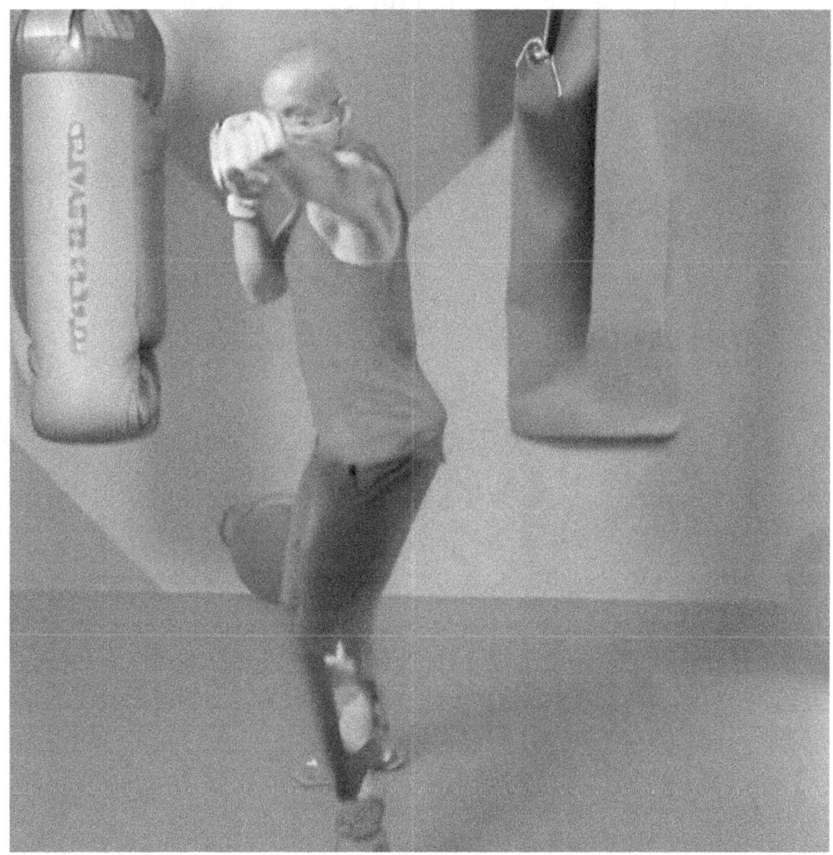

Here are the steps to do this warm up:

1. Stand tall with your shoulder blades back and down, arms at your sides, and feet under your hips.

2. Bring both hands close to your chest, forming fists.

3. Extend your right fist forward, straightening your arm in a punching motion.

4. Bring your right fist back to your chest while extending your left fist forward in a punching motion.

5. Continue this alternating punching motion for the designated time.

Lateral Side Steps

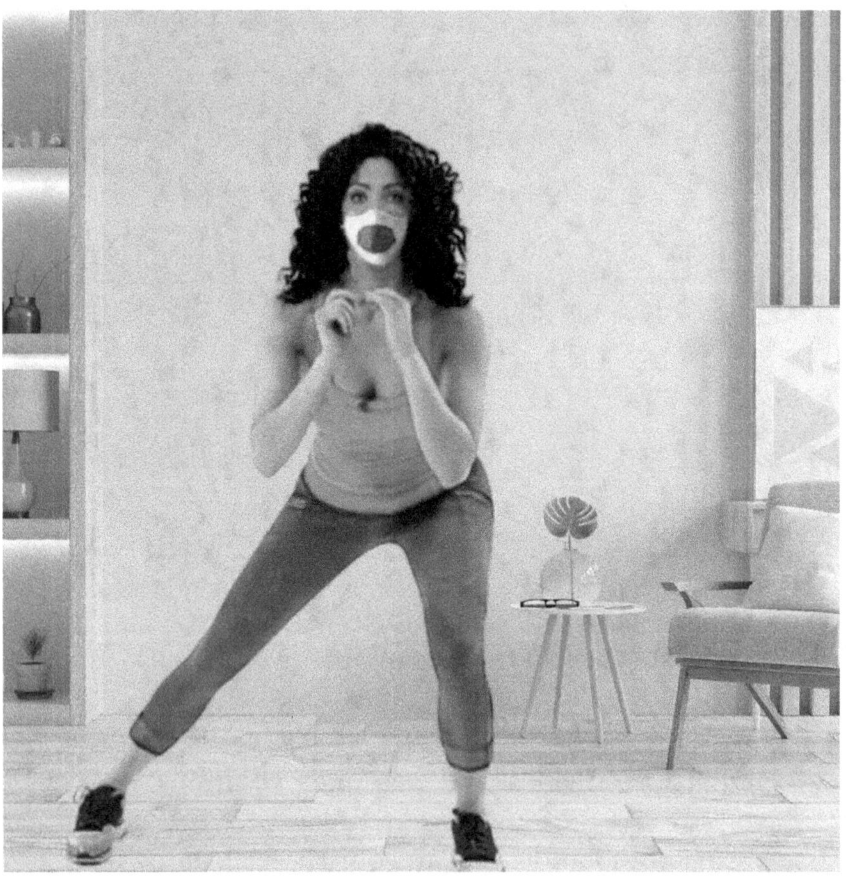

Here are the steps to do this warm up:

1. Stand up tall with your shoulder blades back and down, arms at your sides, and feet under your hips.

2. Bring your hands up to the center of your chest.

3. Bend your knees slightly.

4. Take a lateral step to the left with your left leg.

5. Bring your right leg to meet your left leg so that both feet are together.

6. Take a lateral step to the right with your right leg.

7. Bring your left leg to meet your right leg so that both feet are together.

8. Continue this lateral side-stepping motion for the designated time.

9. Starting with 30 seconds is a good place to begin.

Mobility-Based Warm Up Exercises

Head Rolls

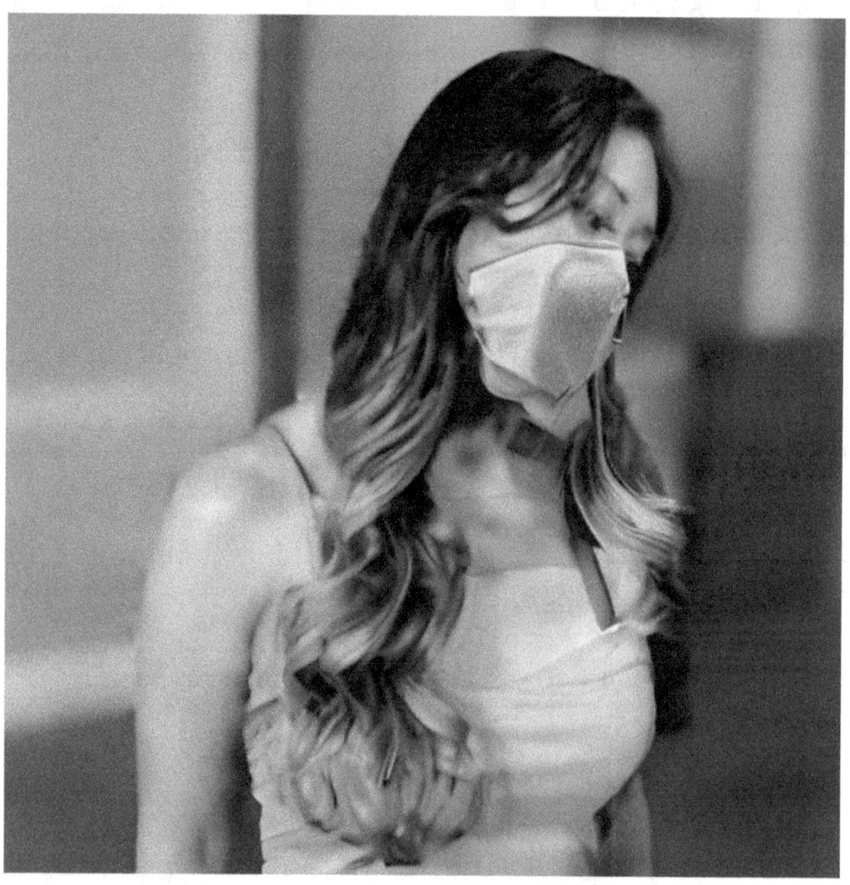

Here are the steps to do this warm up:

1. Stand or sit up tall in a chair with your shoulders down and back.

2. Tuck your chin down towards your chest.

3. Gently roll your head to the left, passing your left shoulder, extending backward, and coming past your right shoulder to return to the starting position.

4. Repeat the head rolls for the required amount of repetitions, typically 10 to 15 reps.

5. Repeat the head rolls in the other direction.

Neck Rotations

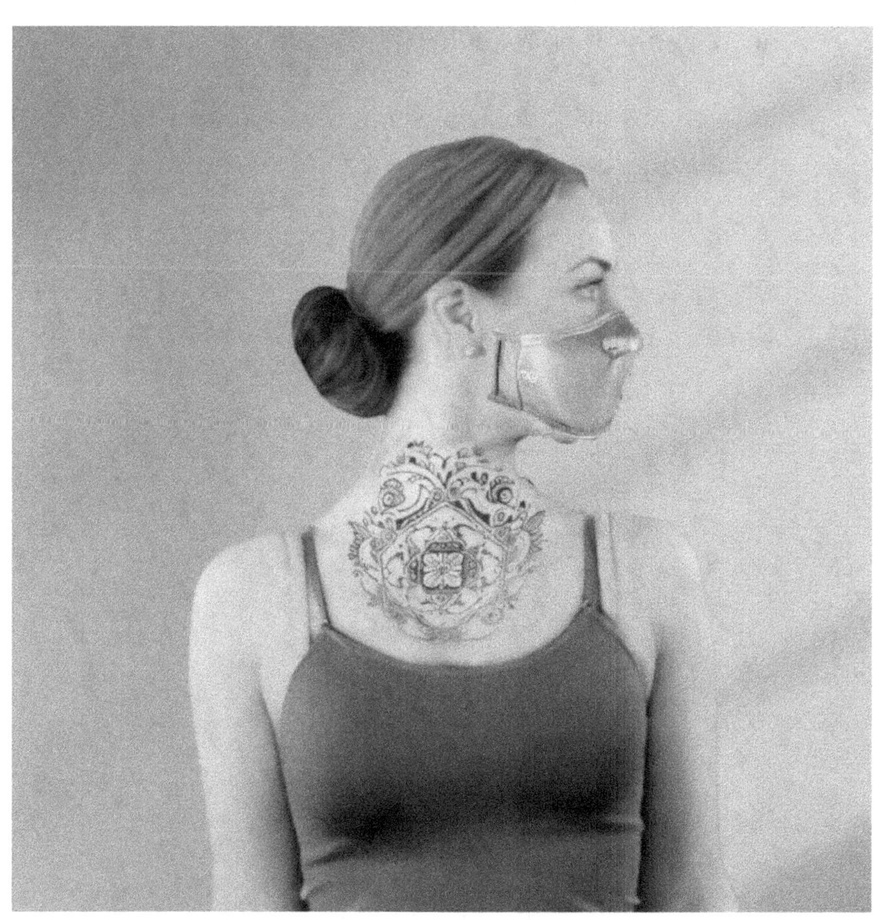

Here are the steps to do this warm up:

1. Stand or sit up tall in a chair with your shoulders down and back.

2. Keeping your torso facing forward and only moving your head, gently turn to look over your right shoulder.

3. Return to the center.

4. Keeping your torso facing forward and only moving your head, gently turn to look over your left shoulder.

5. Repeat the neck rotations for the required amount of repetitions, typically in the range of 10 to 16 reps.

Neck Lateral Flexion

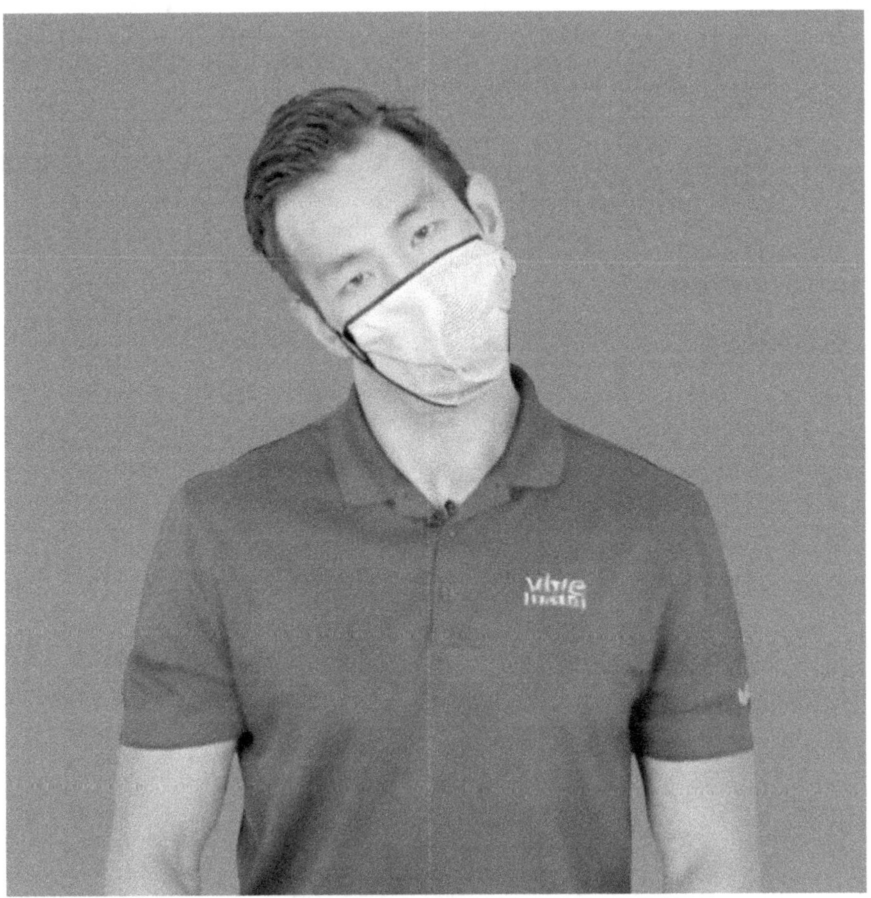

Here are the steps to do this warm up:

1. Stand or sit up tall in a chair with your shoulders down and back.

2. Keeping your torso facing forward, gently bend your right ear towards your right shoulder.

3. Return to the center.

4. Keeping your torso facing forward, gently bend your left ear towards your left shoulder.

5. Repeat the neck lateral flexion for the required amount of repetitions, typically in the range of 10 to 16 reps.

Wrist Rotation

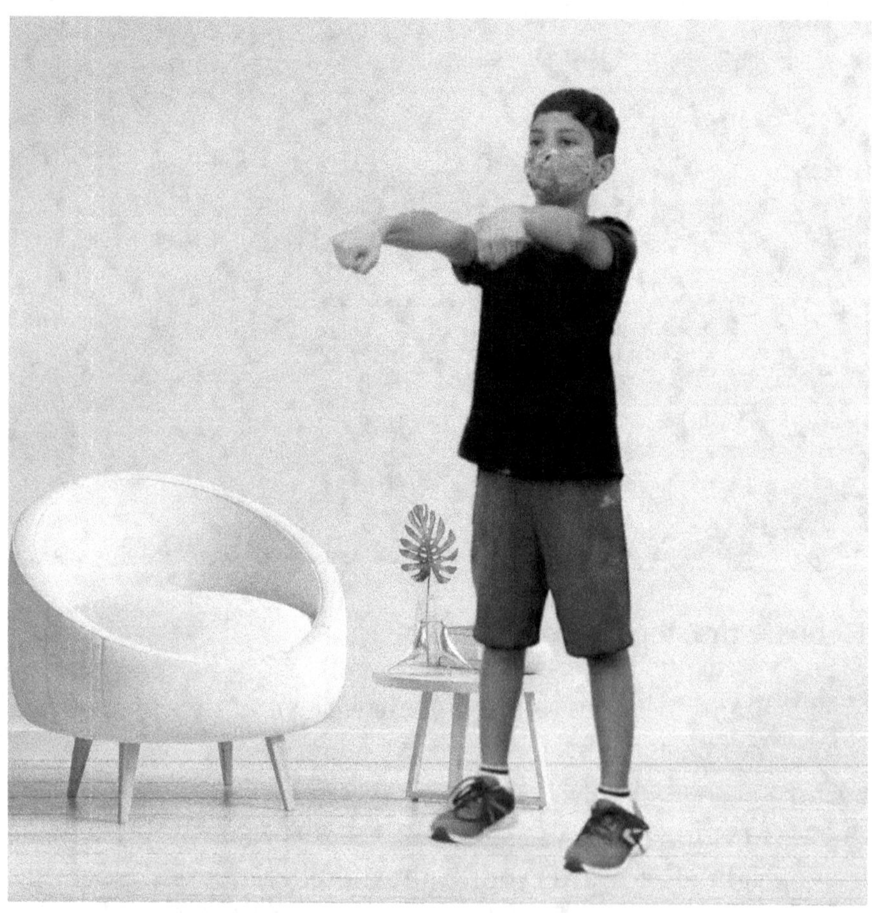

Here are the steps to do this warm up:

1. Start by raising your arms in front of you and clenching your hands into fists.

2. Moving from your wrists, rotate your hands inwards in a circular motion.

3. Repeat the wrist rotations for the required amount of repetitions, typically around 10 reps.

4. Now, rotate your hands outward to repeat the wrist rotations in the opposite direction.

Forearm Circles

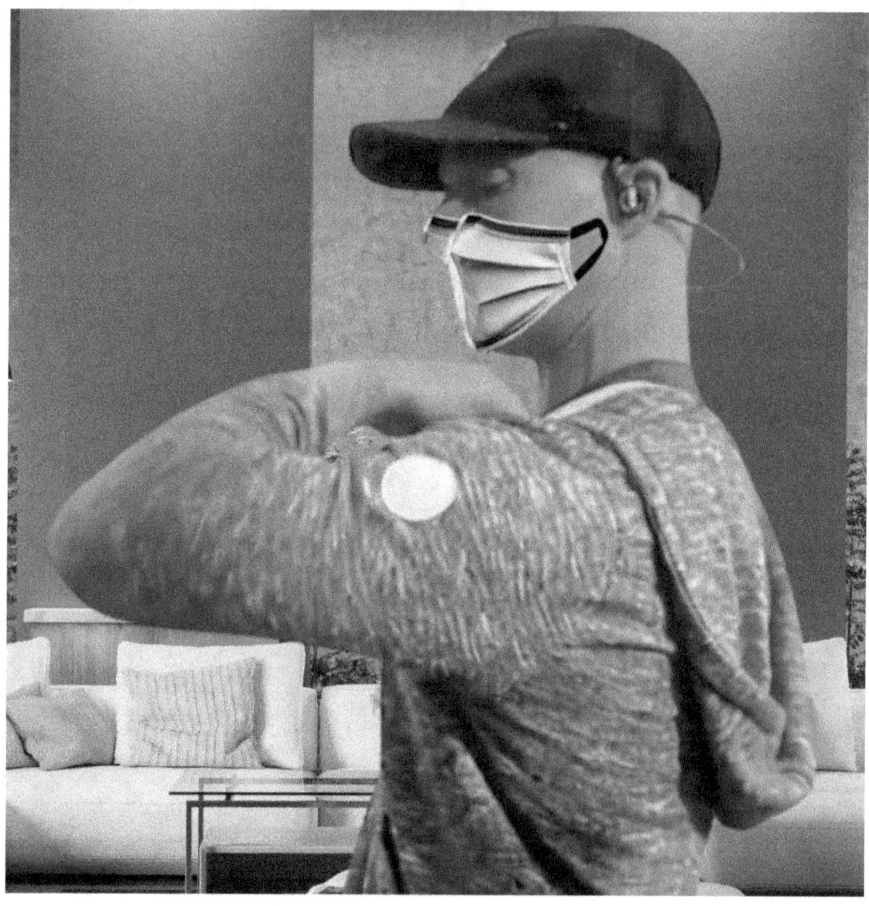

Here are the steps to do this warm up:

1. Start by tucking your elbows into the side of your body, raising your forearms parallel to the floor, with palms facing forward.

2. Moving from your elbows, slowly rotate your forearms forward in circular motions.

3. Repeat the forearm circles for the required amount of repetitions, usually around 10 reps.

4. Now, reverse the direction and repeat the forearm circles in the opposite direction.

Arm Circles

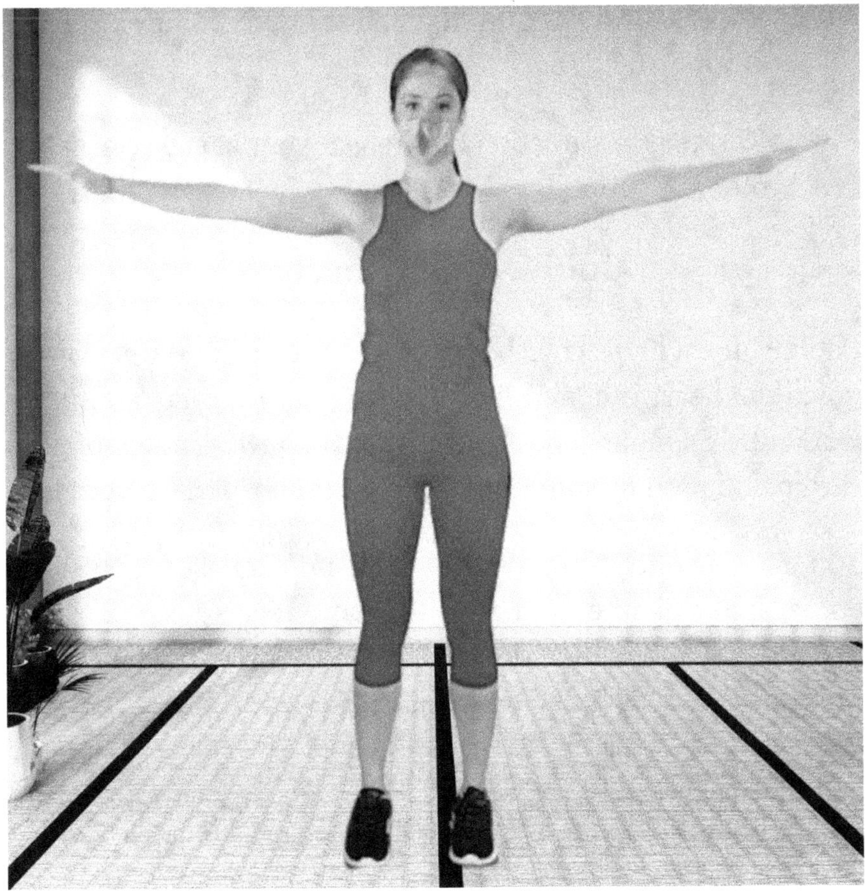

Here are the steps to do this warm up:

1. Stand tall with your shoulders down and back, and your feet under your hips.

2. Straighten your arms out to your sides.

3. Moving from your shoulders, rotate your arms in wide circles forward.

4. Repeat for the required amount of repetitions, typically around 10-15 reps.

5. Reverse the direction and repeat your arm circles in the other direction.

Cool Down Exercises

Cooling down helps your body return to its usual state, slowing down the heart rate and letting your muscles relax after your workout. A simple cool-down involves a few minutes of slow cardio, followed by some stretching or rehab/prehab exercises.

You can use one of the cardio warm-up exercises mentioned earlier in the chapter and do it at a more relaxed pace for your cool-down. Then, include one or two of the stretches and movements below based on the exercises you did that day.

Cat/Cow Stretch

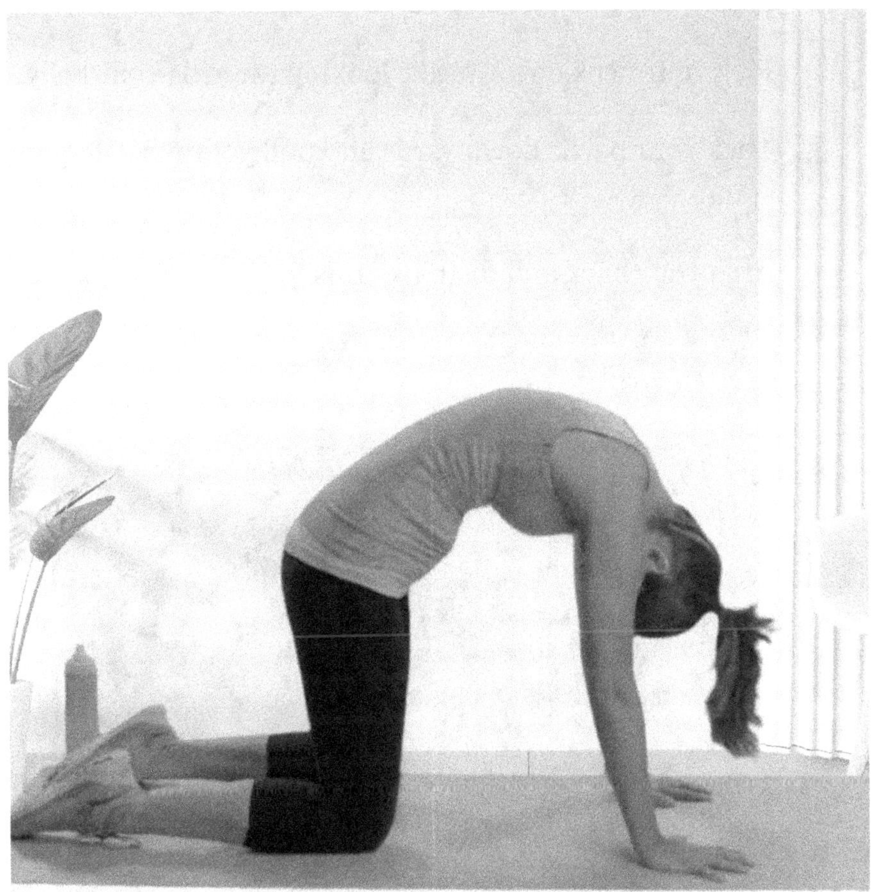

Here are the steps to do this cool down exercise:

1. Start on the floor on all fours, with your hands placed underneath your shoulders and knees underneath your hips.

2. Look upwards towards the ceiling, only moving your neck.

3. Drop your belly towards the ground while tilting your pelvis upwards.

4. Flex your neck downwards, looking towards your belly.

5. Tuck your pelvis downwards and pull your navel to your spine.

6. Arch your back and forth like this for five repetitions.

Forward Bend

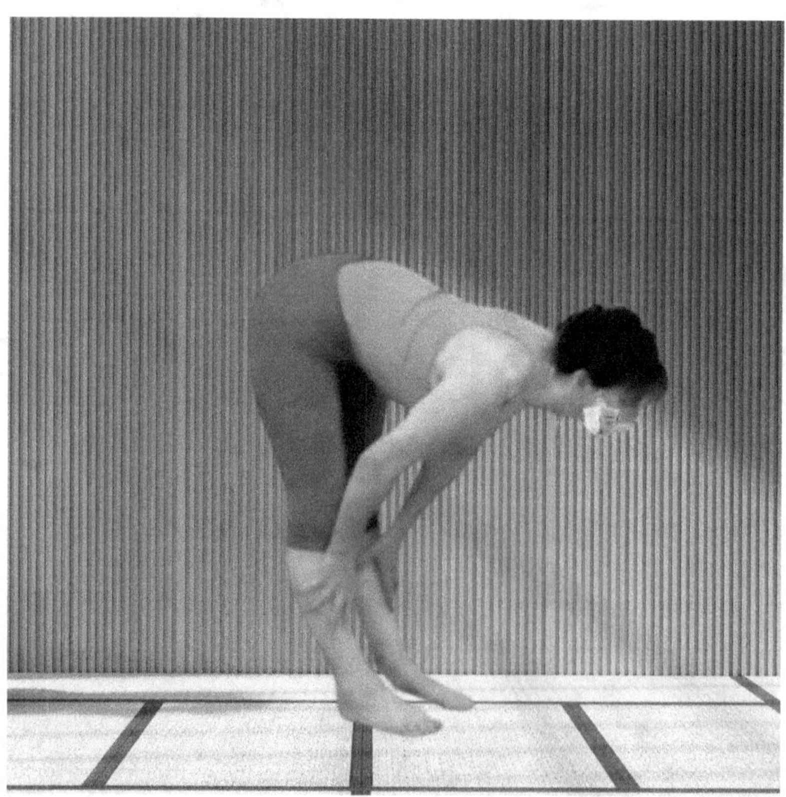

Here are the steps to do this cool down exercise:

1. Stand tall with your shoulders back and down, and your feet placed under your hips.

2. Fold forward gently, hinging from your hips, and reach for your toes.

3. Roll slowly back up, extending your arms over your head and actively reaching for the ceiling.

4. Repeat this sequence for five repetitions.

Hamstring Stretch

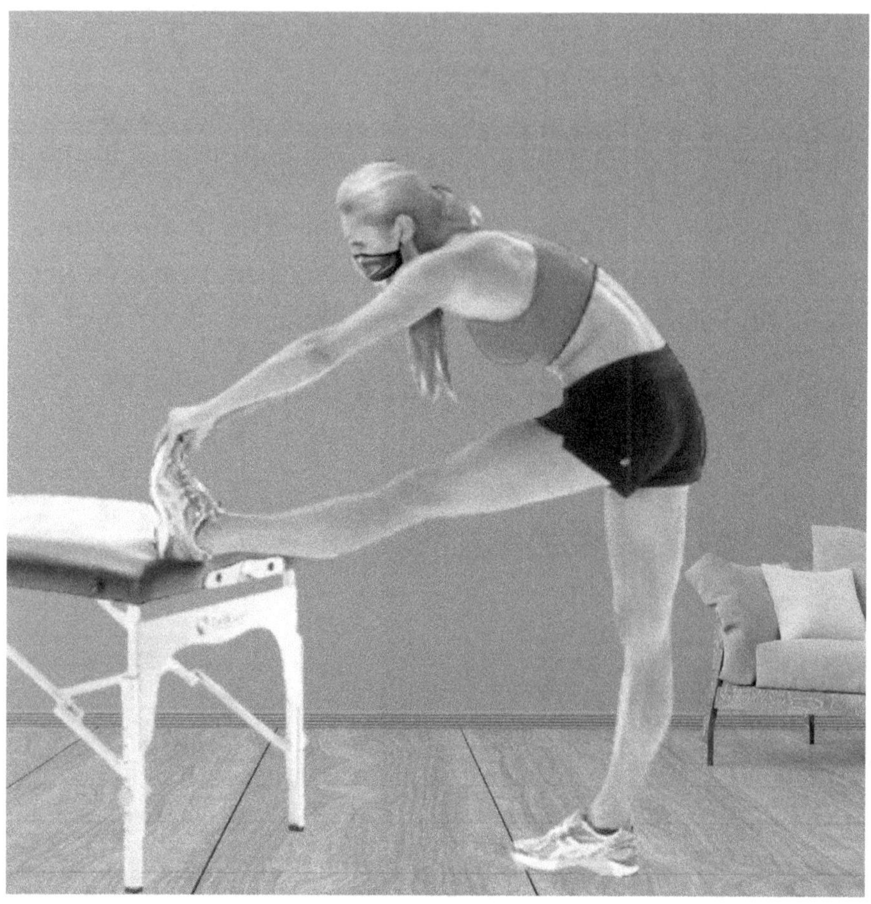

Here are the steps to do this cool down exercise:

1. Stand tall with your shoulders back and down, and your feet placed under your hips. You can use a chair to help keep you balanced.

2. Keeping one leg straight, place that foot in front of you while keeping both heels on the ground.

3. Ensure the toes of your back leg face forward and soften your knee.

4. Keep your back straight and your hips facing forward as you lean towards your front leg.

5. Feel the stretch in the back of your leg.

6. Hold the stretch for the set time.

7. Swap legs and repeat.

Quadruped Stretch

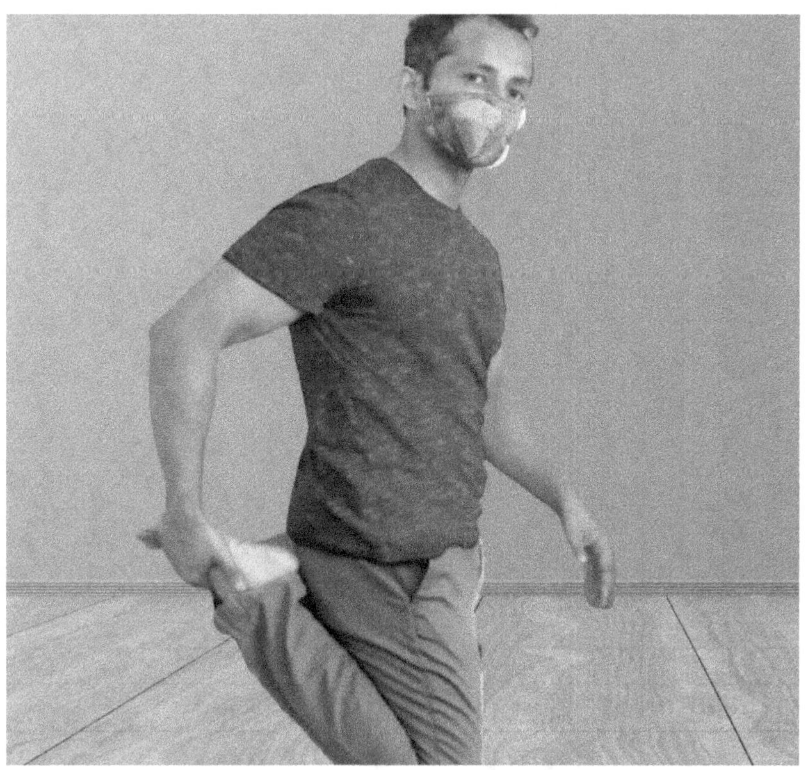

Here are the steps to do this cool down exercise:

1. Stand tall with your shoulders back and down, and your feet placed under your hips. You can use a chair to help keep you balanced.

2. Holding onto your foot, bring your left leg up and behind you, pulling your heel towards your glutes.

3. Keep your back straight and upright, and ensure your knees are together.

4. Hold the stretch for a set amount of time.

5. Swap legs and repeat.

Calf Stretch

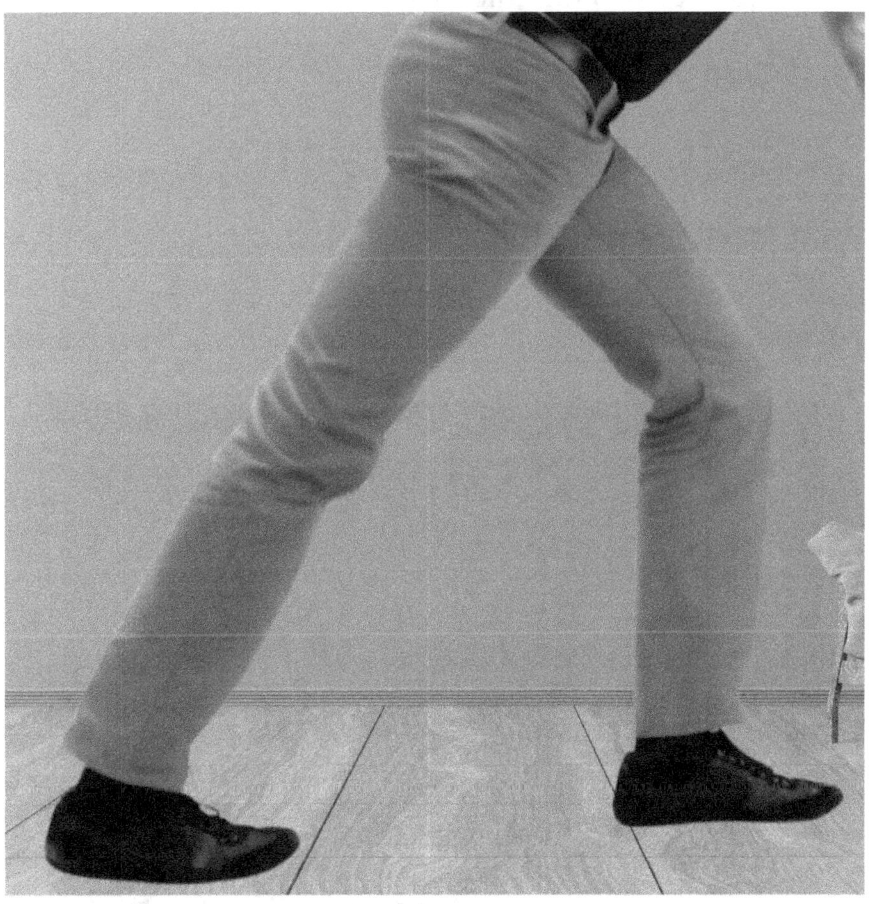

Here are the steps to do this cool down exercise:

1. Stand tall with your shoulders back and down, and your feet placed under your hips. Hold onto the back of a chair for balance.

2. Keep your toes facing forward and take a step back with your right leg.

3. Keep your heels on the ground and gently bring your front knee toward the chair.

4. Lean gently into the stretch.

5. Hold the stretch for a set amount of time.

6. Swap legs and repeat.

Abductor Stretch

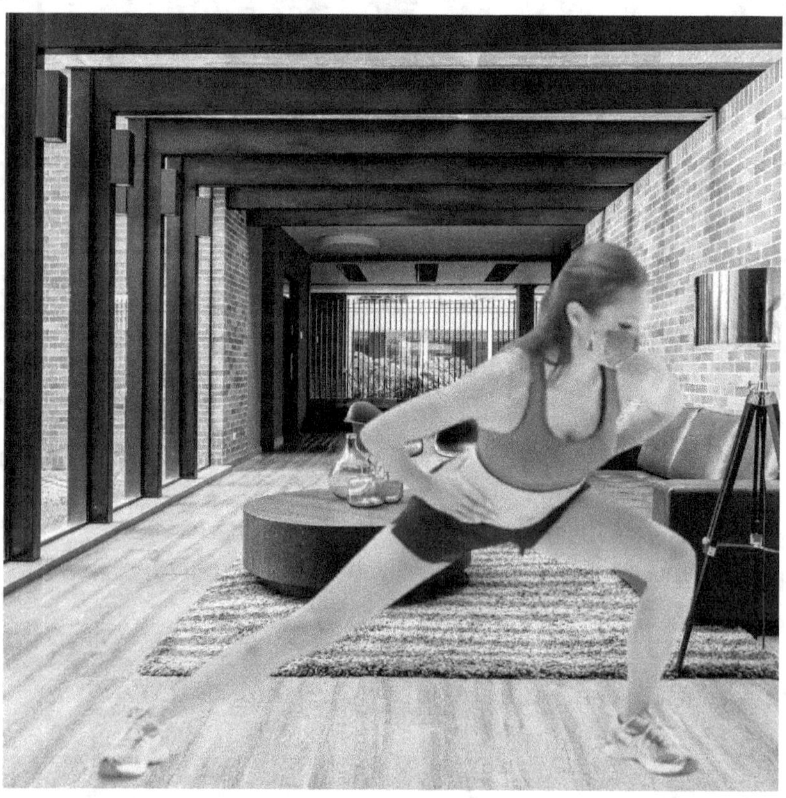

Here are the steps to do this cool down exercise:

1. Stand tall with your shoulders back and down, and your feet placed under your hips.

2. Step your right leg out to the side, keeping both feet with their toes pointing forward or slightly out to the side.

3. Gently bend your right leg and shift your weight onto it, keeping your left leg straight as you lean.

4. Keep your left foot planted firmly on the ground.

5. Feel the stretch in your inner thigh.

6. Hold the stretch for a short amount of time.

7. Swap legs and repeat.

CHAPTER 3: RESISTANCE BAND EXERCISES

This chapter will serve as your exercise library. I've gathered a bunch of resistance band movements and organized them into three sections:

- Upper body

- Lower body

- Full body

You can do many of these exercises while sitting or using a chair for support. When picking the right resistance band, go for one that makes your muscles feel moderately to very tired after doing 20–30 reps. If you can do 20 reps without much effort, the band is too easy. On the other hand, if you can only manage 2–4 reps, it's too light.

Here are some important things to keep in mind while doing your exercises:

- Don't hold your breath; remember to breathe.

- Exhale when you're doing the toughest part of the exercise.

- Do your movements slowly and with control.

- Make sure to use the full range of motion for each joint and muscle you're working on.

Upper Body Exercises

Band Pull Aparts

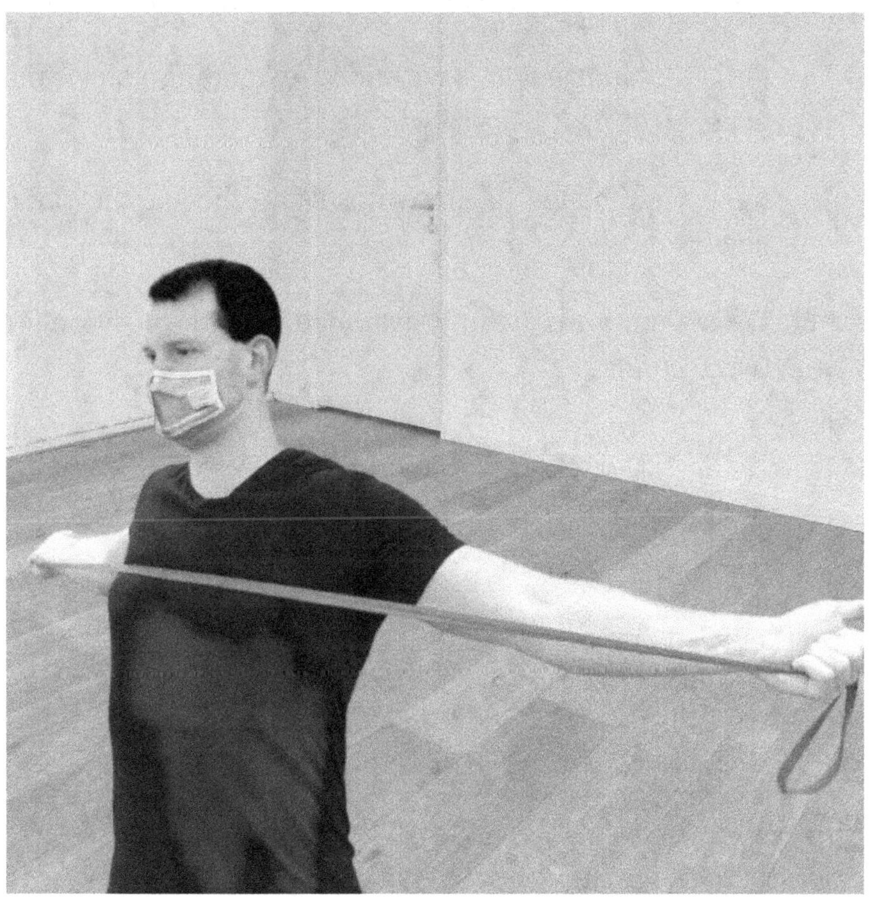

Here are the steps to do this exercise with resistance band:

1. Stand tall with your shoulders back and down, and your feet underneath your hips.

2. Hold the end of the resistance band in each hand.

3. Lift your arms straight in front of you until they reach shoulder height, with your palms facing downward. Maintain a slight tension in the band, but not too tight.

4. Pull the band out to your sides, extending your arms wide, creating a T position.

5. Keep your hands in line with each other at the same height.

6. When your arms are fully extended, hold the position for two seconds.

7. Return to the center.

8. Repeat for the recommended reps, with the average being 10 repetitions.

Bow and Arrow

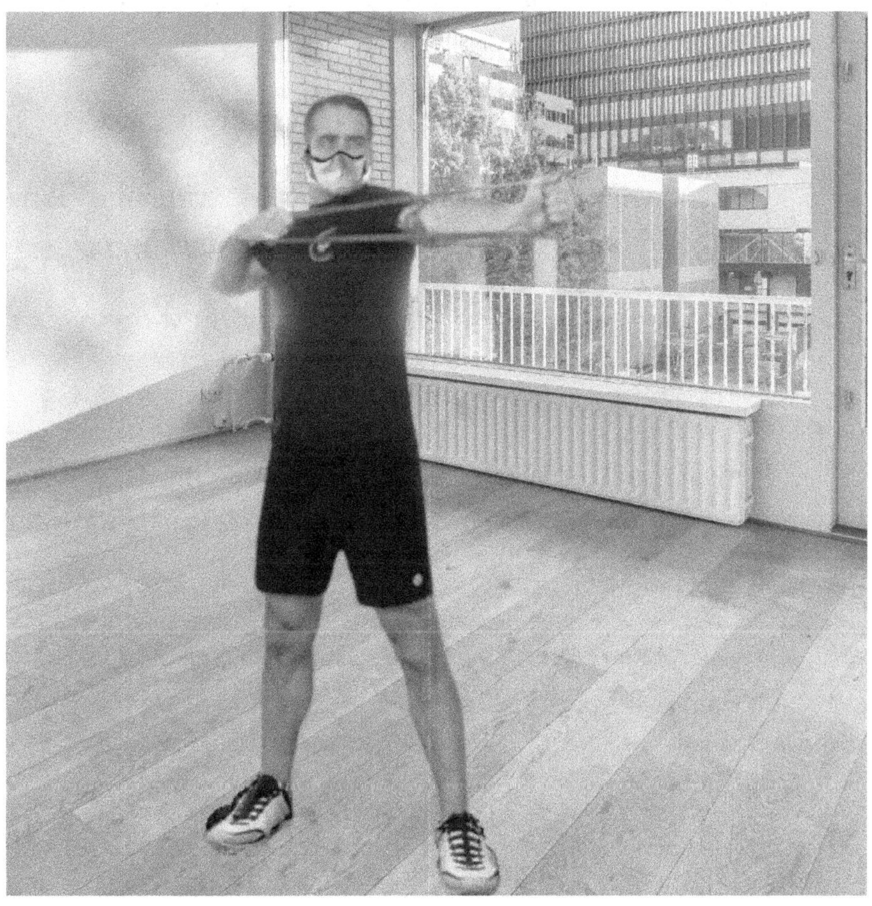

Here are the steps to do this exercise with a resistance band:

1. Stand tall with your shoulders back and down, feet underneath your hips, and engage your core.

2. Hold the end of the resistance band in each hand.

3. Raise both hands to chest level.

4. Find your starting position by extending your left arm to your left side while keeping your right arm in line with the middle of your chest.

5. Adjust the band tension so there's light resistance.

6. Pull your right hand away from your left arm, mimicking the motion of drawing back an arrow from a bow.

7. Keep your elbows elevated and pointed outwards.

8. Return to the starting position.

9. Repeat for the recommended reps on one side, then switch to the other. The average is 10-12 repetitions per side.

Lateral Raise

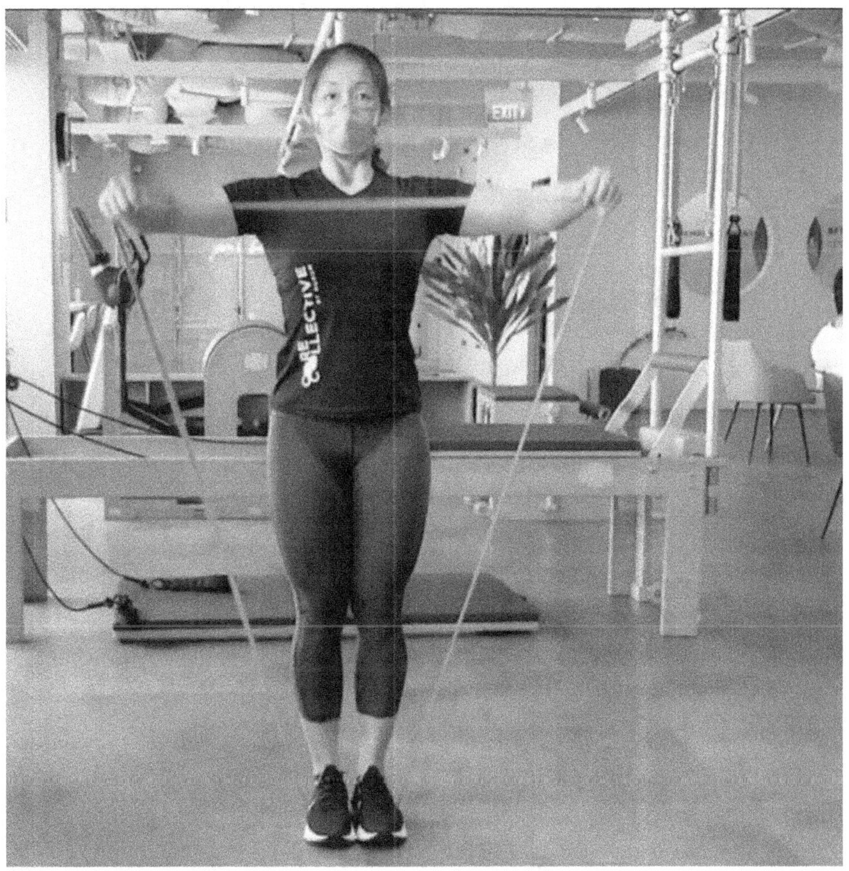

Here are the steps to do this exercise with a resistance band:

1. Stand tall with your shoulders back and down, and place your feet underneath your hips.

2. Hold the end of the resistance band in each hand and loop it under both your feet.

3. Keep your arms straight, then raise them to your side until they align with your shoulder blades.

4. Return to the starting position.

5. Repeat for the recommended amount of reps. The average is 10-15 repetitions.

Staggered Stance Row

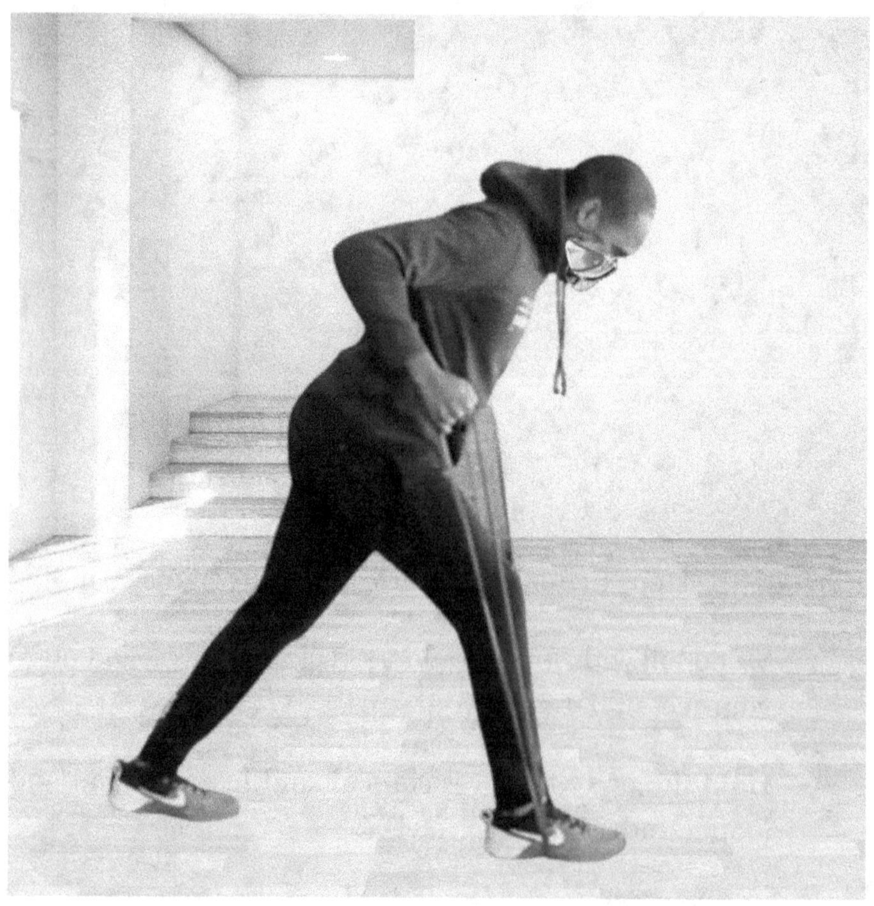

Here are the steps to do this exercise with a resistance band:

1. Stand up tall with your shoulders back and down.

2. Place your left foot in front of your right, creating a staggered stance. Widen your stance slightly for better balance.

3. Hold the end of the resistance band in each hand and loop it under your left foot.

4. Bend your left leg slightly, engage your core, and lean forward from your hips while maintaining a straight back.

5. Extend your arms down toward your left foot to set up the starting position, ensuring the band has light tension.

6. Pull your hands towards your torso in a rowing motion, keeping your elbows, arms, and hands in line with your ribcage.

7. Complete the rep by extending your arms back to the starting position.

8. Repeat for the recommended reps on one side, then switch feet. The average is 8-12 repetitions per side.

Bent Over Row

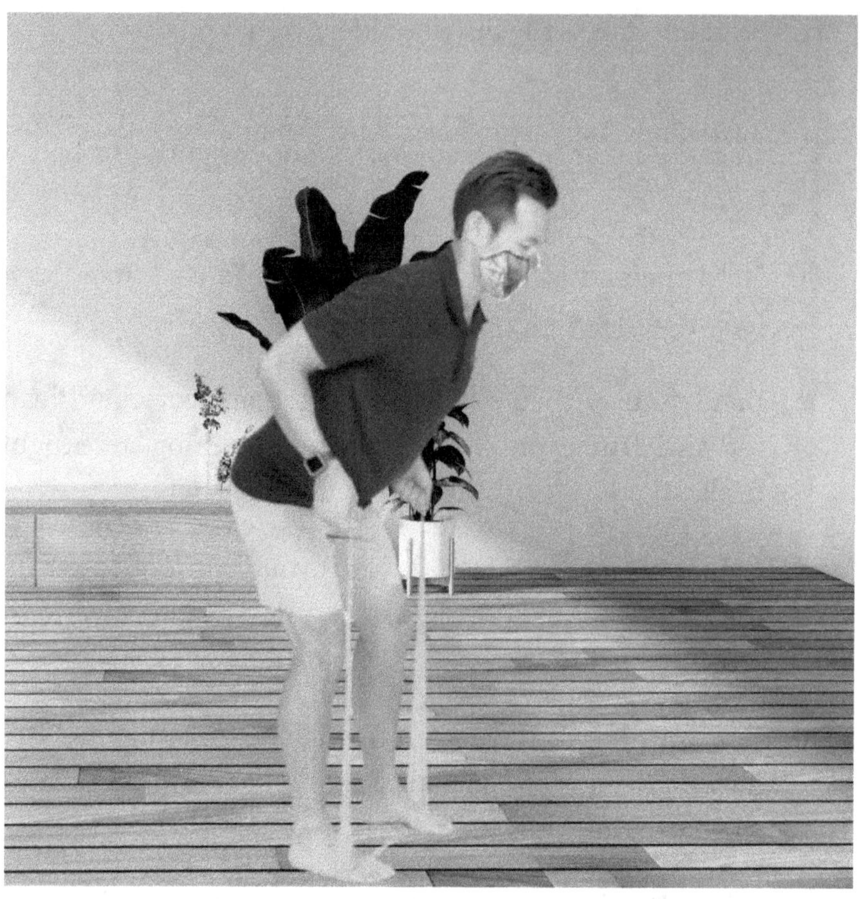

Here are the steps to do this exercise with a resistance band:

1. Stand up tall with your shoulders back and down. Position your feet underneath your hips.

2. Hold the end of the resistance band in each hand and loop it under both of your feet.

3. Bend forward from your hips, lowering your upper body until it's parallel to the floor.

4. Allow your arms to lower towards your feet, maintaining a straight back.

5. Initiate the movement by pulling your arms towards your ribcage squeezing your shoulder blades together. Ensure your elbows point up towards the ceiling.

6. Return to the starting position.

7. Repeat for the recommended amount of reps. The average is 10–15 repetitions.

Seated Row

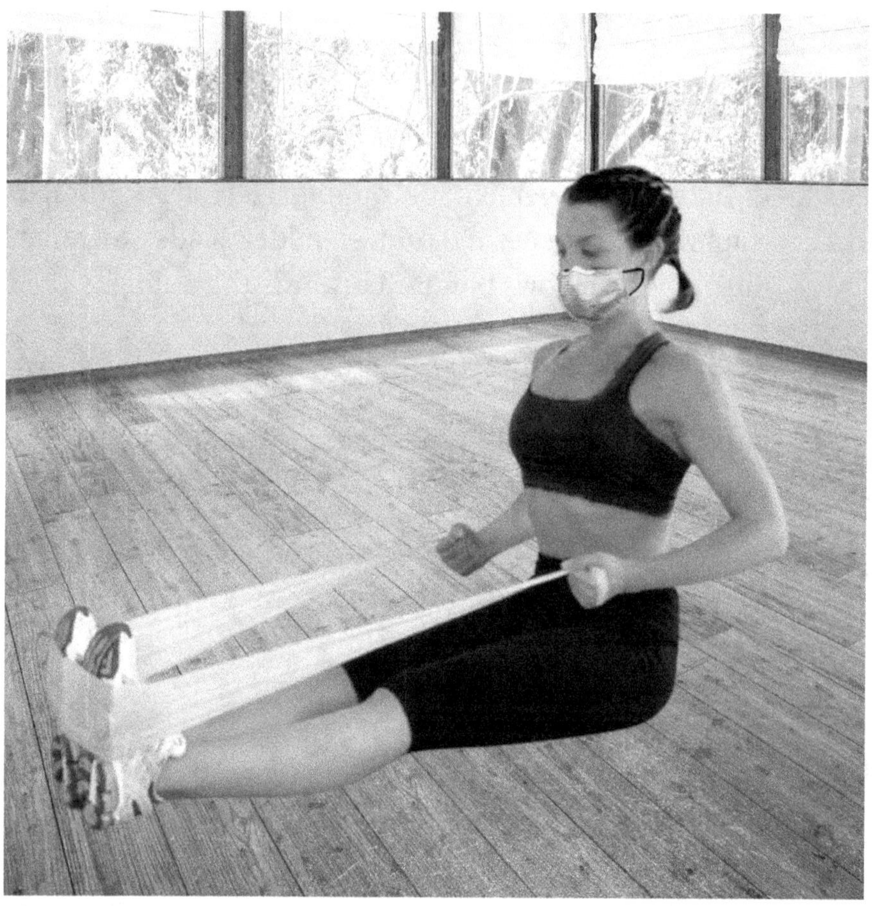

Here are the steps to do this exercise with a resistance band:

1. Sit on the floor with your legs stretched out in front of you.

2. Loop the resistance band around the soles of your feet, holding each end of the band with your palms facing each other.

3. Bend your knees slightly.

4. Pull the band towards your navel by keeping your back straight and elbows close to your sides.

5. When your arms reach a 90° angle, squeeze your shoulder blades together.

6. Slowly return to the starting position.

7. Repeat for the recommended amount of reps. The average is 10–15 repetitions.

Banded Front Raise

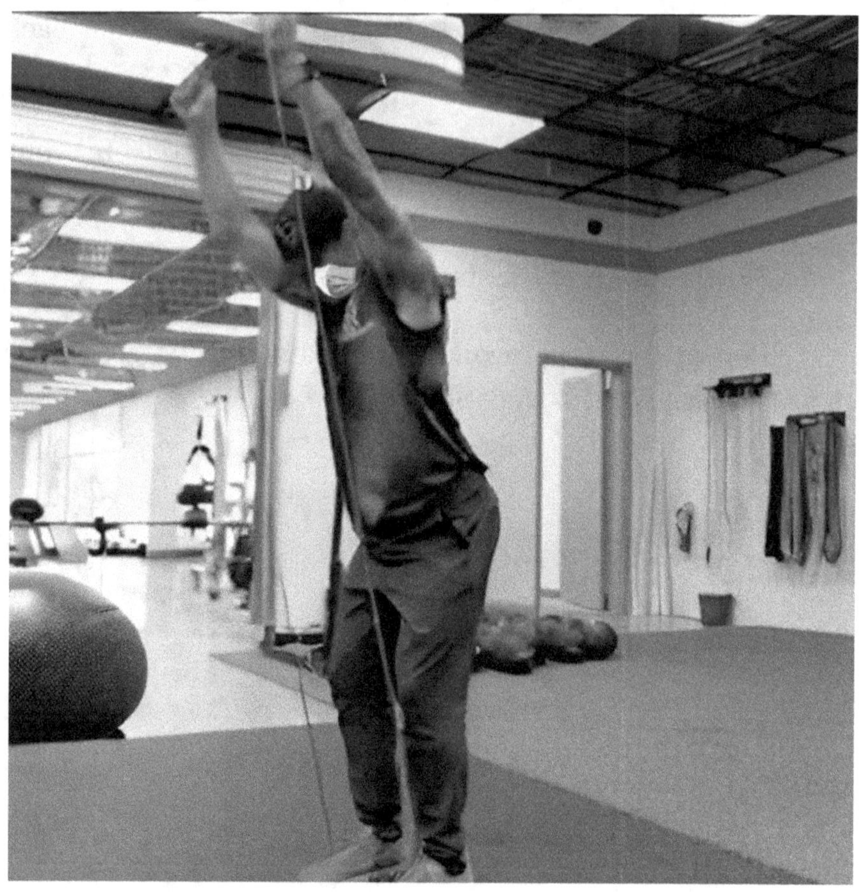

Here are the steps to do this exercise with a resistance band:

1. Stand tall with your shoulders back and down, feet underneath your hips.

2. Hold the end of the resistance band in each hand, looping it under both of your feet.

3. Pull the band up in front of you, keeping your arms straight.

4. Stop when you reach shoulder height.

5. Return to the starting position.

6. Repeat for the recommended amount of reps. The average is 10–15 repetitions.

Cuff Pivot

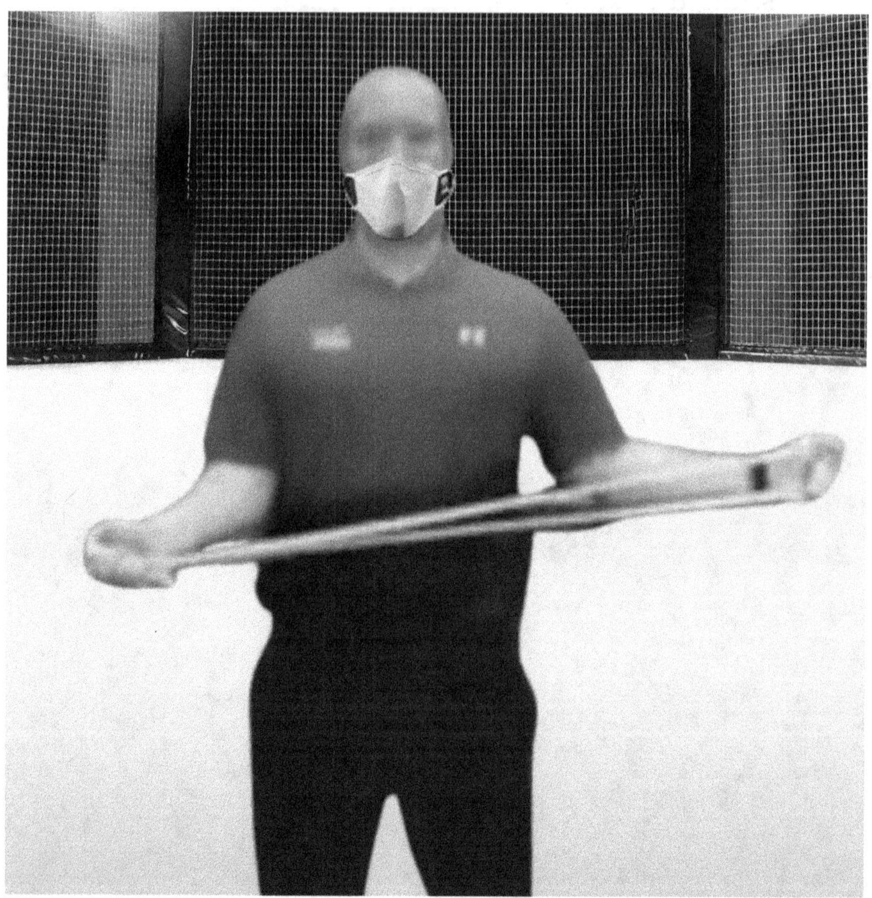

Here are the steps to do this exercise with a resistance band:

1. Stand up tall with your shoulders back and down, engaging your core.

2. Hold each end of the resistance band in your hands, just below your chest and in line with the bottom of your ribcage.

3. Bend your elbows and point them outwards.

4. If you have a short band, great! If not, wrap it around your hand a few times to create tension.

5. Keep your left hand still and pull your right hand outwards, maintaining a fixed elbow at your waist.

6. Focus on rotating your arm using your shoulder blades, keeping your arm bent.

7. Return to the starting position and repeat on the same side for the recommended reps. The average is 10–12 reps on one side.

Chest Press

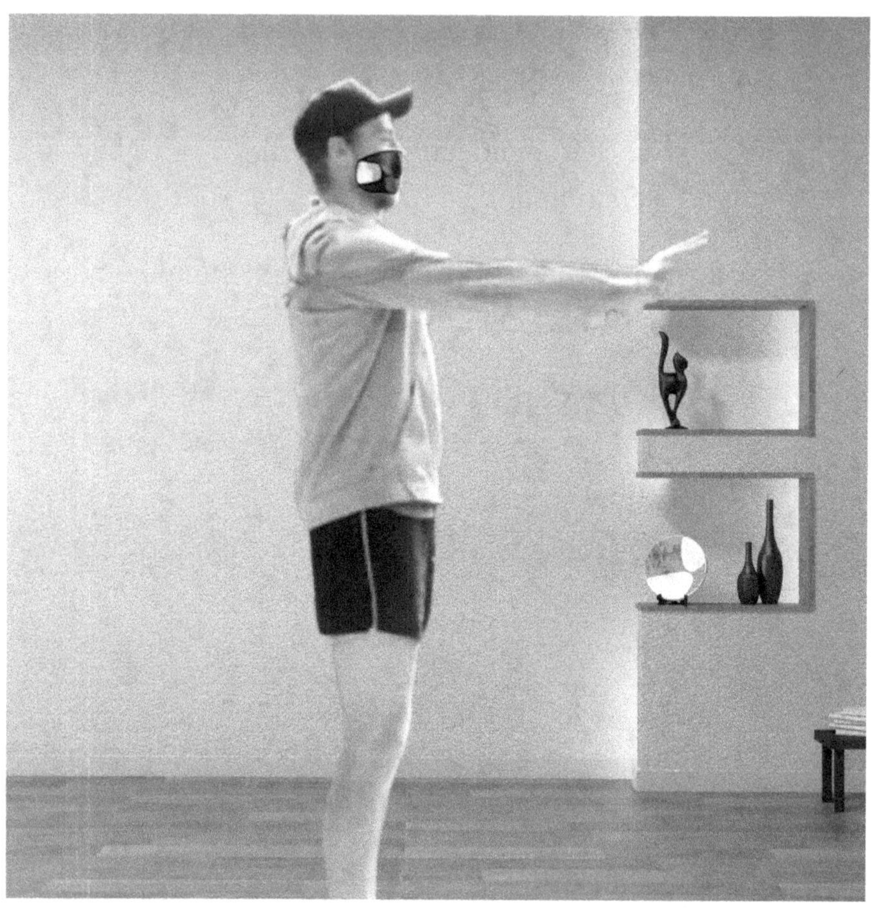

Here are the steps to do this exercise with a resistance band:

1. Stand up tall with your shoulders back and down, engaging your core.

2. Hold each end of the resistance band in your hands and place the middle section behind your upper back, in line with your shoulders.

3. Extend your arms in front of you with the palms facing downward.

4. Return to the starting position.

5. Repeat for the recommended amount of reps. The average is 10–15 repetitions.

Scapular Retraction

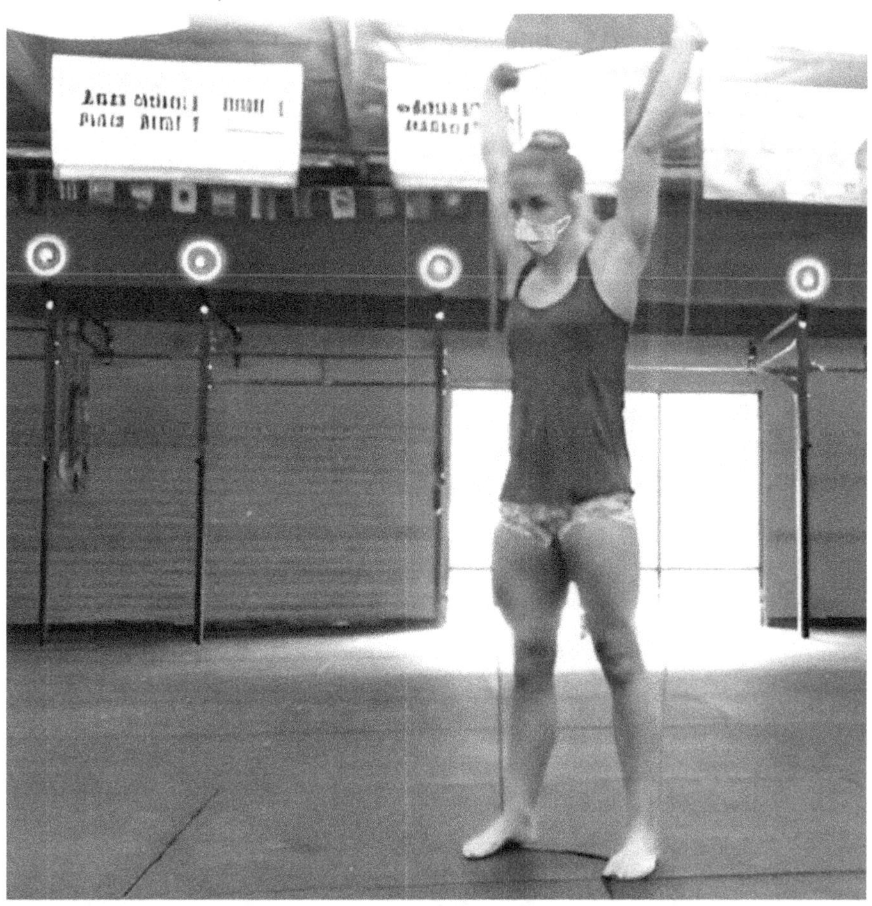

Here are the steps to do this exercise with a resistance band:

1. Stand tall with your shoulders down and back, ensuring your feet are underneath your hips.

2. Place the resistance band around your wrists, adjusting the length as needed.

3. With palms facing forward and fingers pointing to the ceiling, position your arms at a 90° angle.

4. Slowly rotate your elbows out while squeezing your shoulder blades together.

5. Keep your core tight and maintain a straight back throughout the movement.

6. Pause and squeeze your shoulder blades together for two seconds.

7. Release and return to the starting position.

8. Repeat for the recommended amount of reps. The average is 10–15 repetitions.

Overhead Press

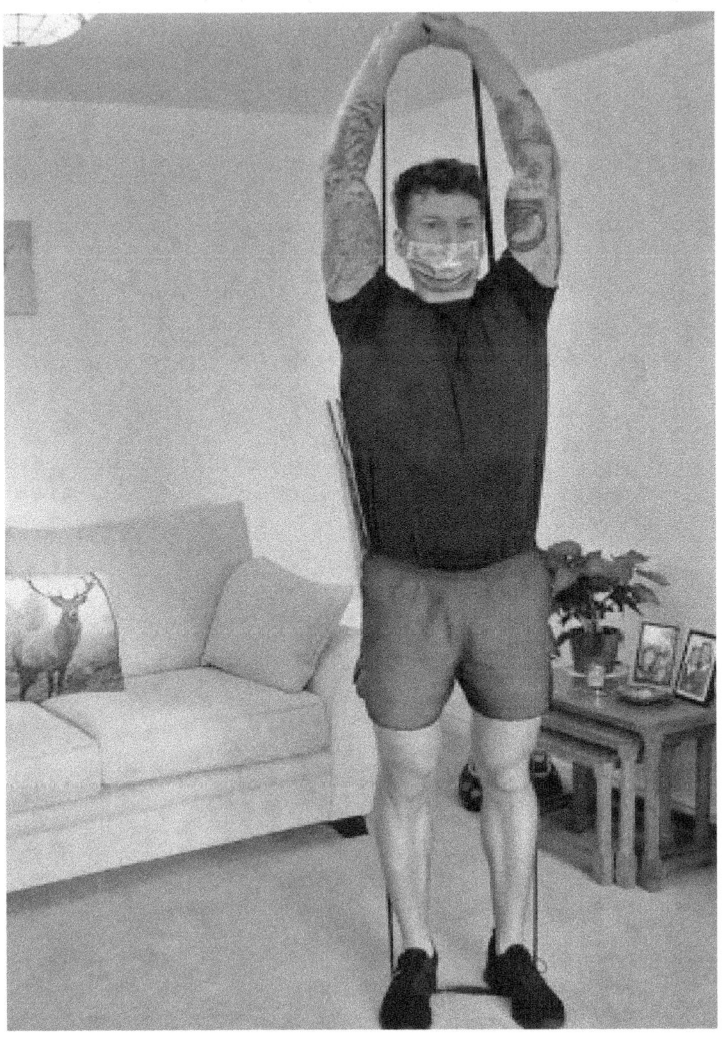

Here are the steps to do this exercise with a resistance band:

1. Stand tall with your shoulders down and back, ensuring your feet are underneath your hips.

2. Loop the resistance band underneath both of your feet, holding each end of the band in one hand at shoulder height. Palms should be facing forward.

3. Press your arms straight up over your head, avoiding arching backward. Keep your back straight throughout the movement.

4. Lower your arms back down to your collarbone.

5. Repeat for the recommended amount of reps. The average is 8–12 repetitions.

Overhead Triceps Extension

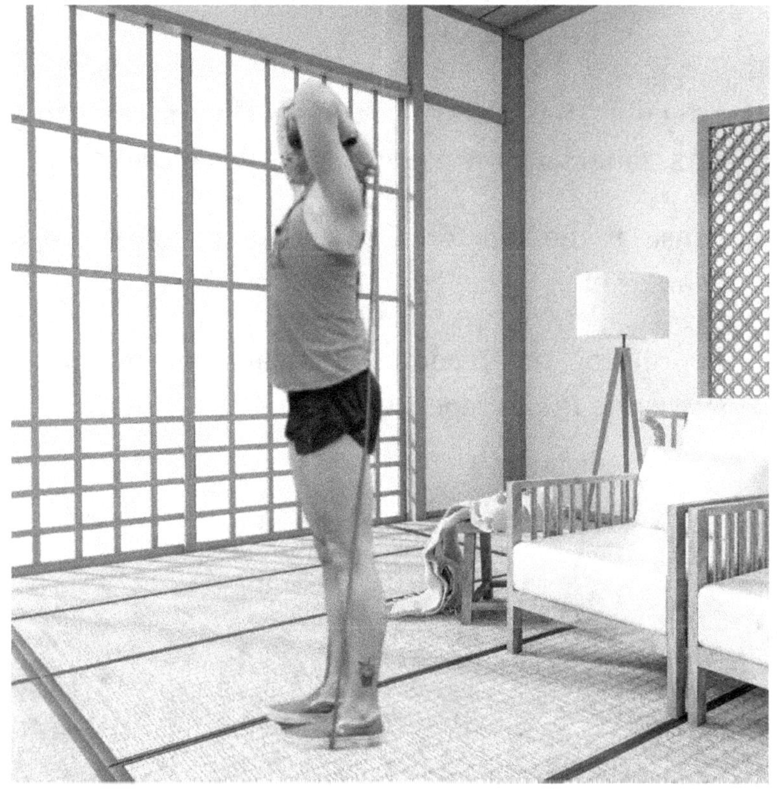

Here are the steps to do this exercise with a resistance band:

1. Stand tall with your shoulders down and back, ensuring your feet are close together.

2. Loop the resistance band underneath both feet and hold each end of the band behind your head, running along your back.

3. Start with your elbows close to your ears, palms facing each other, and knuckles touching.

4. Straighten your elbows without moving your arms, extending them overhead. Keep elbows close to your ears, shoulders down, and engage your core.

5. Pause at the top for a second, then lower the band behind you.

6. Repeat for the recommended amount of reps. The average is 15–20 repetitions.

Overhead Pull Apart

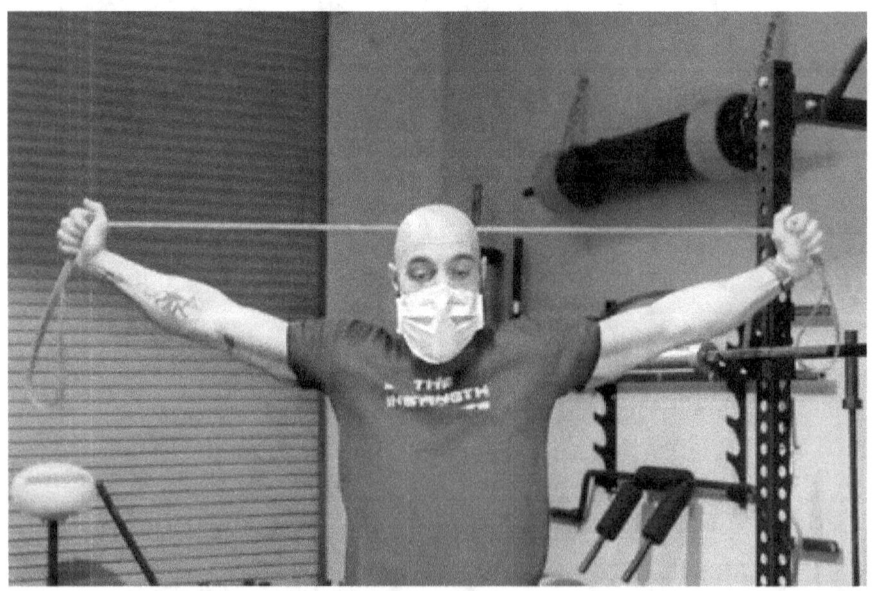

Here are the steps to do this exercise with a resistance band:

1. Stand tall with your shoulders down and back, maintaining a shoulder-width stance.

2. Hold the ends of the resistance band in each hand and raise your arms overhead, directly above you.

3. As you bring the band down behind your back, simultaneously pull it apart, stretching it across your shoulders with your hands fully extending to either side.

4. Hold this stretched position for a second before slowly returning to the starting position.

5. Repeat for the recommended amount of reps. The average is 8–12 repetitions.

Biceps Curl

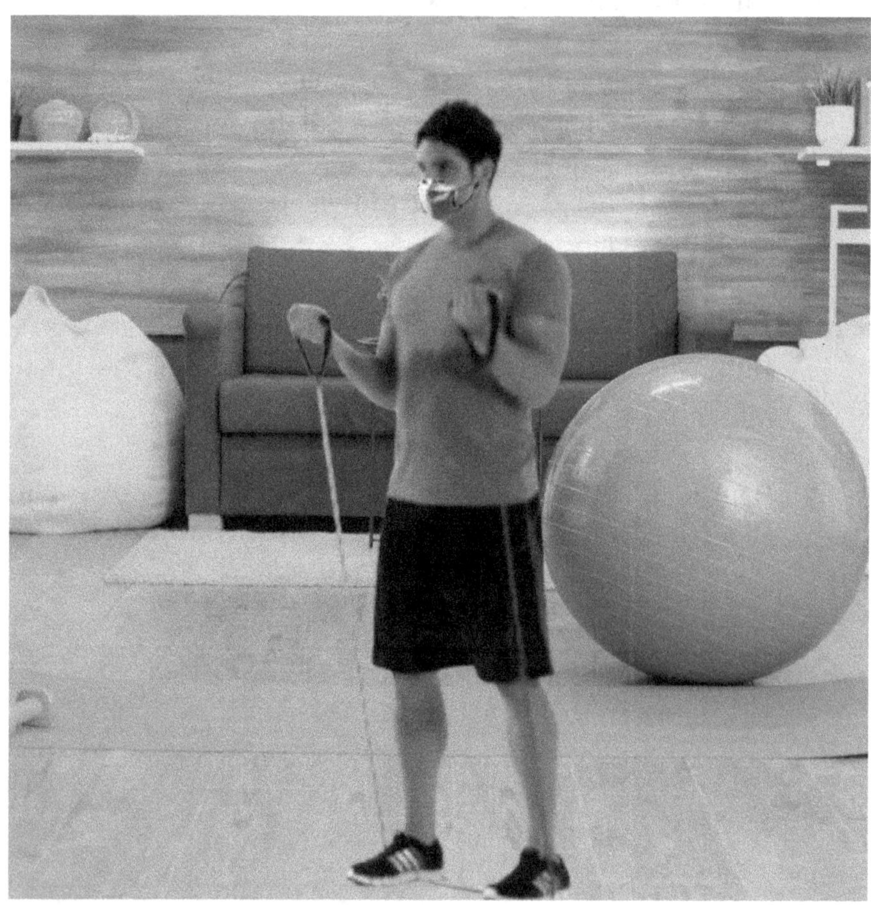

Here are the steps to do this exercise with a resistance band:

1. Stand tall with your shoulders down and back, ensuring your feet are underneath your hips.

2. Loop the resistance band underneath both feet, holding each end of the band in one hand with your palms facing forward. Allow your arms to hang by your sides.

3. Bend your elbows, slowly curling your hands towards your shoulders, squeezing your biceps. Keep your elbows close to the sides of your body.

4. Lower your hands back to the starting position.

5. Repeat for the recommended amount of reps. The average is 15–20 repetitions.

Bent Over Rear Dealt Fly

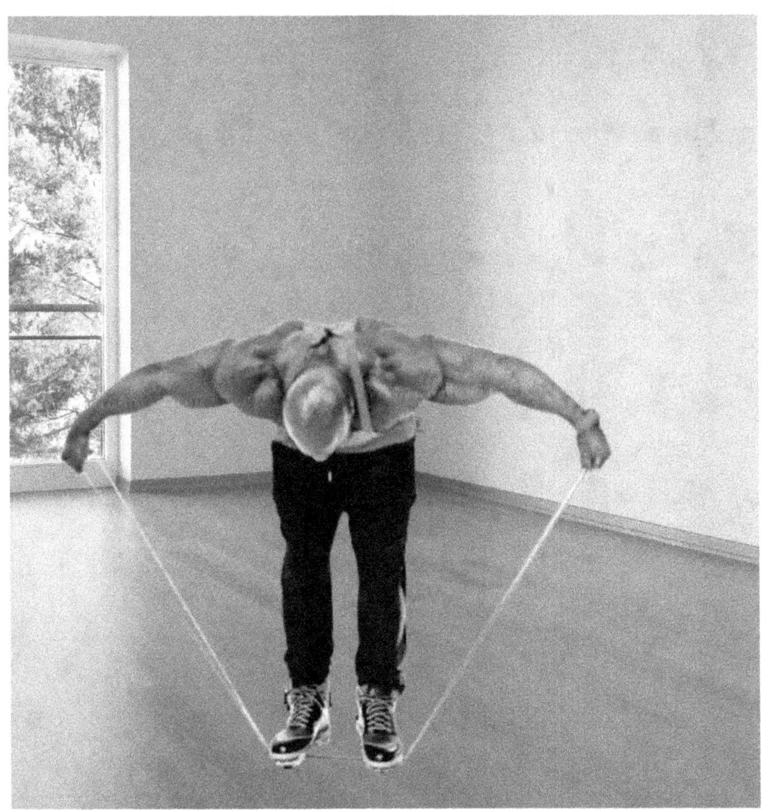

Here are the steps to do this exercise with a resistance band:

1. Stand tall with your shoulders down and back, ensuring your feet are underneath your hips.

2. Loop the resistance band underneath both of your feet, holding each end of the band in one hand with your palms facing each other. Bend forward from your hips, keeping your back straight.

3. Raise your arms straight to your side until you reach shoulder height, squeezing your shoulder blades together.

4. Lower your arms back to the starting position.

5. Repeat for the recommended amount of reps. The average is 10–12 repetitions.

Upright Row

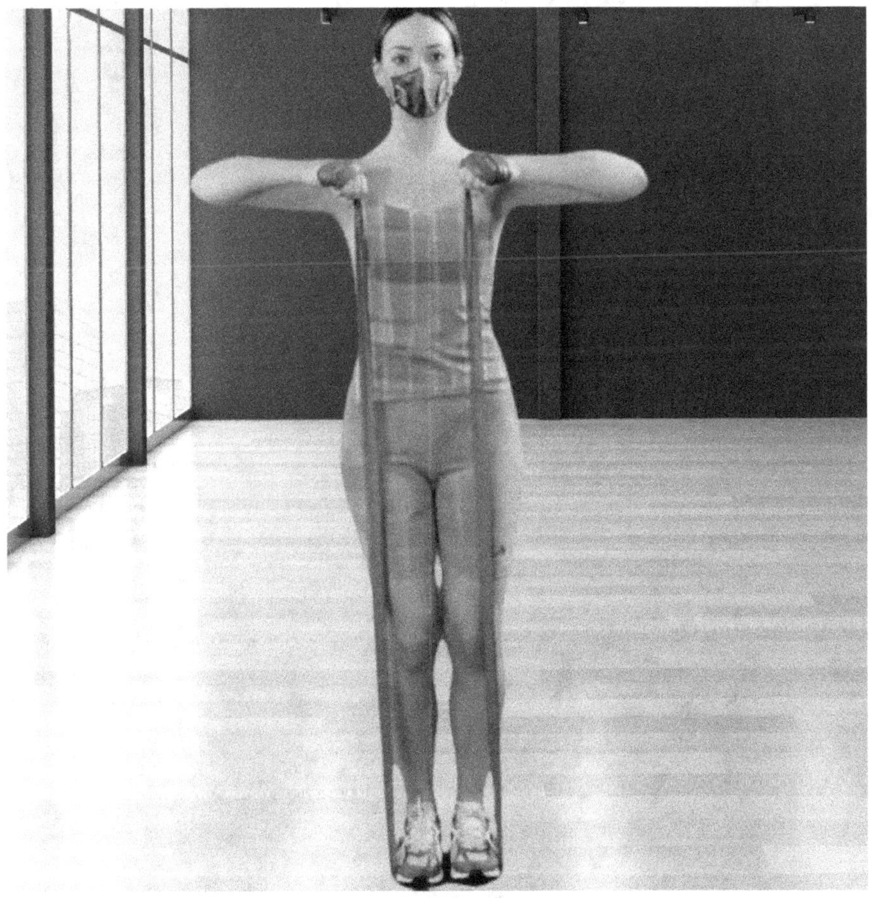

Here are the steps to do this exercise with a resistance band:

1. Stand tall with your shoulders down and back, ensuring your feet are underneath your hips.

2. Loop the resistance band underneath both feet, holding each end of the band in one hand with your palms facing towards you.

3. Bending at the elbows, pull the band straight up the front of your body to shoulder level.

4. Slowly lower back to the starting position.

5. Repeat for the recommended amount of reps. The average is 10–12 repetitions.

Lower Body Exercises

Banded Squat #1

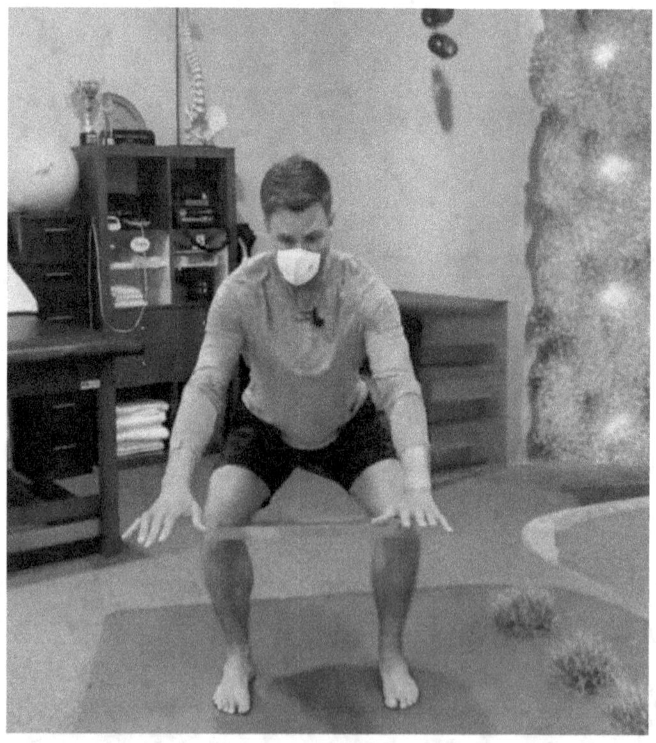

Here are the steps to do this exercise with a resistance band:

1. Stand up tall with your shoulders back and down, engaging your core.

2. Place your feet shoulder-width apart, toes turned slightly outwards.

3. Hold the end of the resistance band in each hand and loop it under both feet.

4. Create tension by pulling the band up towards the middle of your body.

5. Start the squat by pushing your hips back and bending your knees as if sitting down.

6. Keep your back straight and knees driving outwards, staying over your toes.

7. Stand up to return to the starting position.

8. Repeat for the recommended amount of reps. The average is 10–15 repetitions.

Banded Squat #2

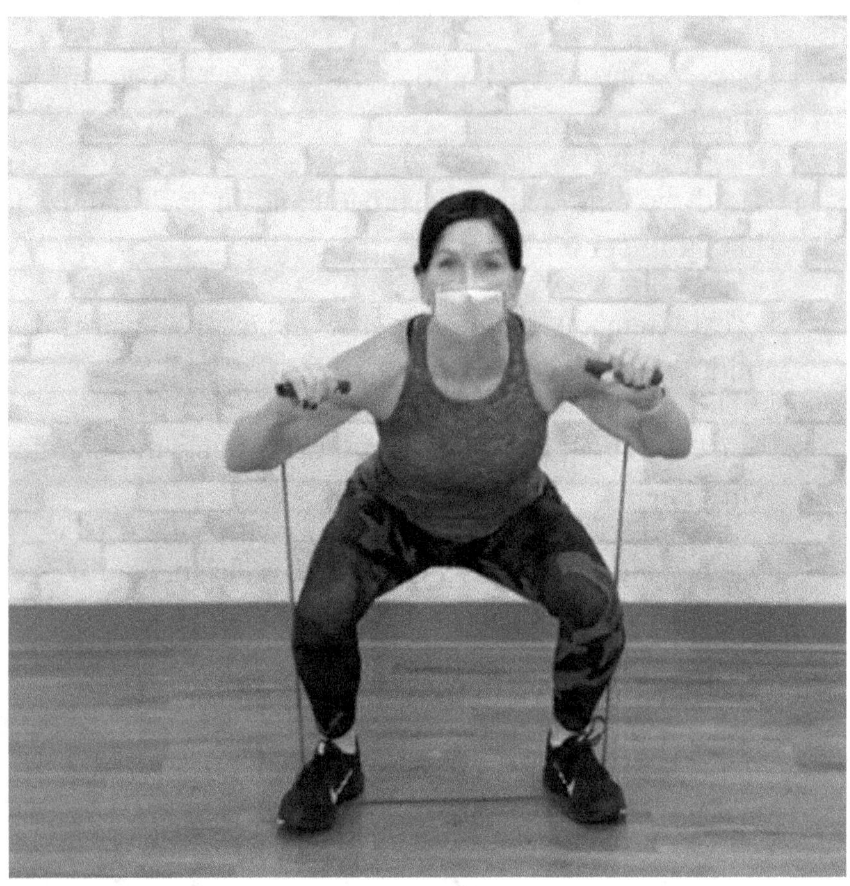

Here are the steps to do this exercise with a resistance band:

1. Stand up tall with your shoulders back and down, engaging your core.

2. Place the resistance band above your knees.

3. Position your feet shoulder-width apart with toes slightly turned outwards.

4. Begin the squat by pushing your hips back and bending your knees as if sitting down.

5. Keep your back straight and ensure your knees are driving outwards over your toes.

6. Stand up to return to the starting position.

7. Repeat for the recommended amount of reps. The average is 10–15 repetitions.

Deadlift

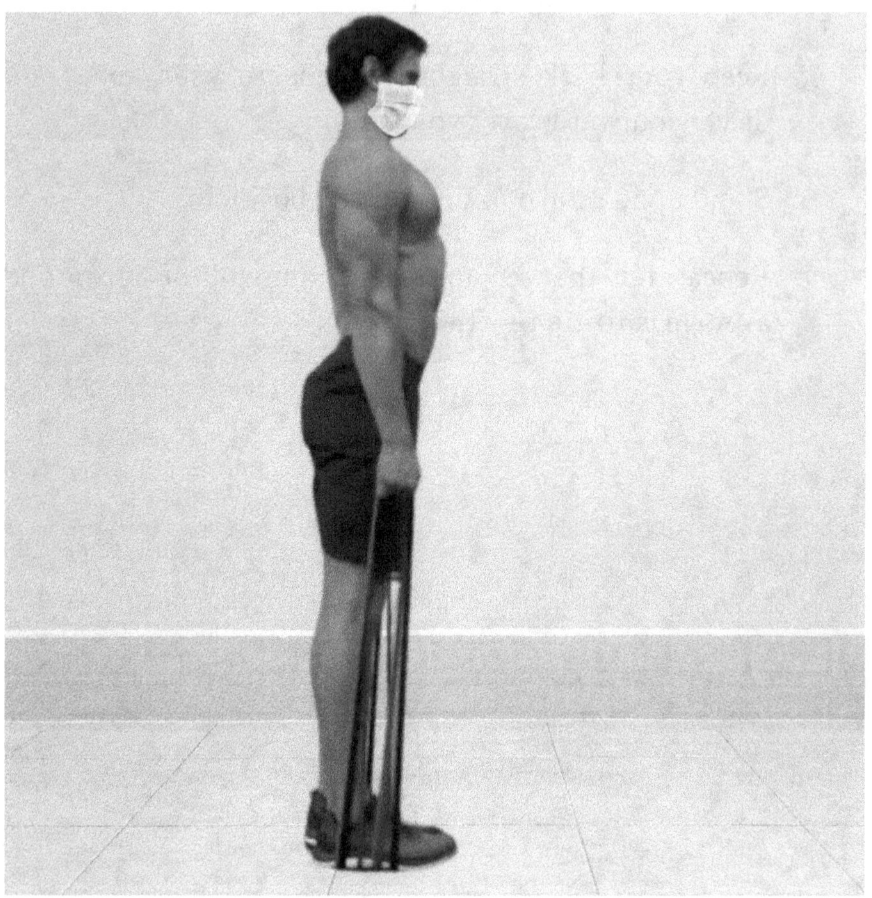

Here are the steps to do this exercise with a resistance band:

1. Stand tall with your shoulders down and back, placing your feet hip-distance apart.

2. Loop the resistance band underneath both feet and hold the other end with both hands.

3. Keep your arms straight and shift your hips backward, entering a hinge position.

4. Lower your torso until it is parallel to the floor, maintaining a straight back.

5. Stand up straight, squeezing your glutes at the top.

6. Repeat for the recommended amount of reps. The average is 10–15 repetitions.

Kickstand Single-Leg-Romanian Deadlift

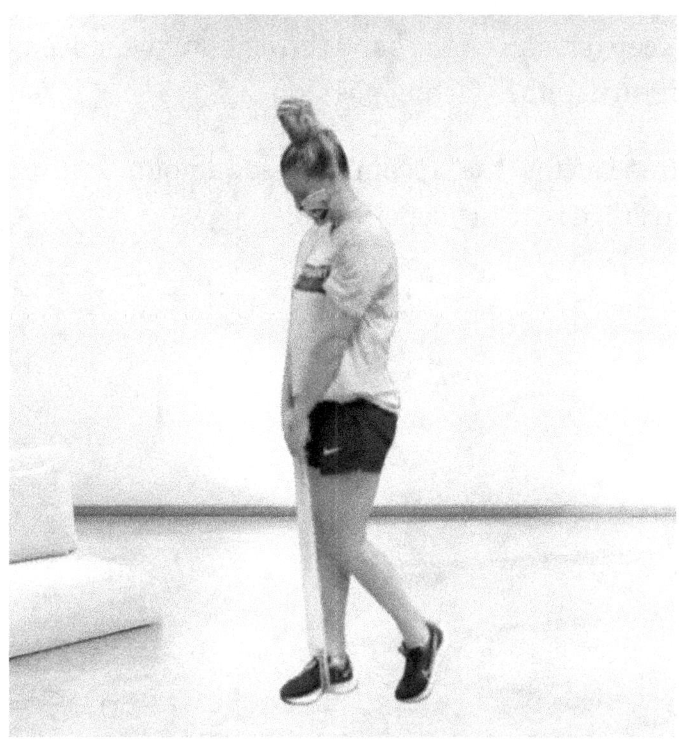

Here are the steps to do this exercise with a resistance band:

1. Stand up tall with your shoulders back and down.

2. Place your right foot in front of your left, creating a staggered stance. Keep your left foot on its ball, adjusting your stance for balance.

3. Hold the end of the resistance band in each hand and loop it under your right foot.

4. Bend your left leg slightly, engage your core, and hinge forward from your hip while maintaining a straight back.

5. Keep tension on the band throughout the movement and return to the starting position.

6. Repeat for the recommended amount of reps. The average is 10–15 repetitions.

Standing Adduction

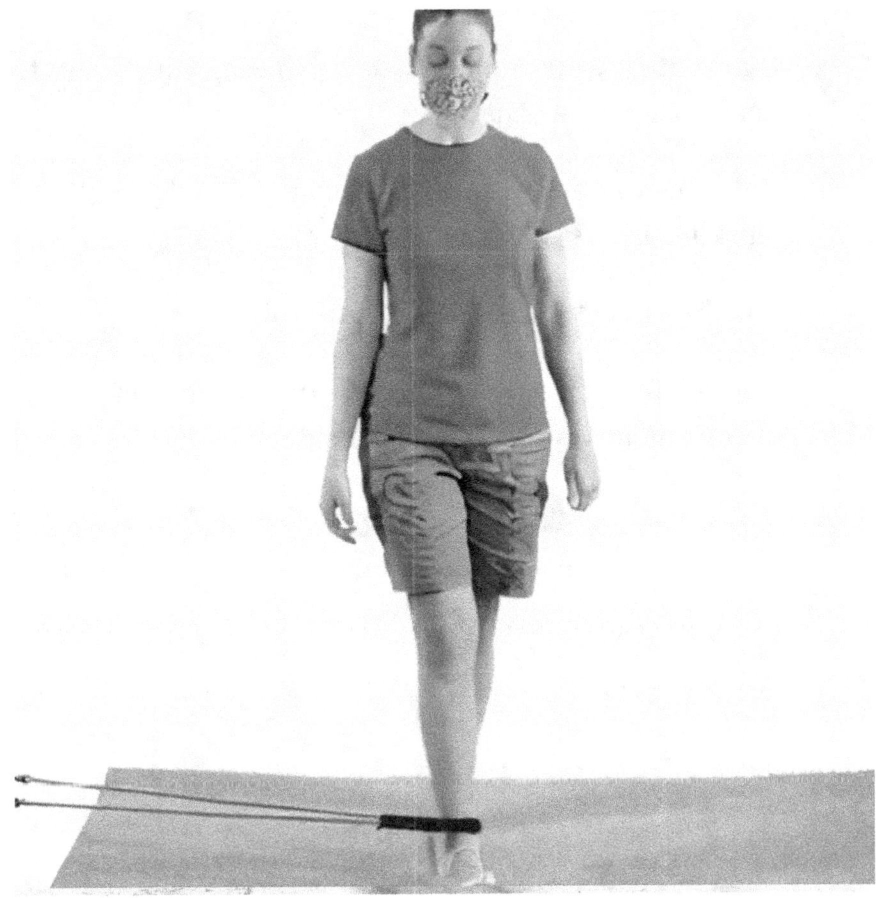

Here are the steps to do this exercise with a resistance band:

1. Anchor the resistance band at ankle height and stand tall, aligning yourself with the band.

2. Wrap the free end of the band around your outer ankle.

3. Stand perpendicular to the band, creating tension by moving away from it.

4. Start with a wide stance, slightly bending your knees to get into a partial squat.

5. Pull your outer leg in toward your inner leg, actively working against the band's resistance.

6. Slowly return to the starting position.

7. Repeat for the recommended amount of reps. The average is 12–15 repetitions per side.

Leg Press

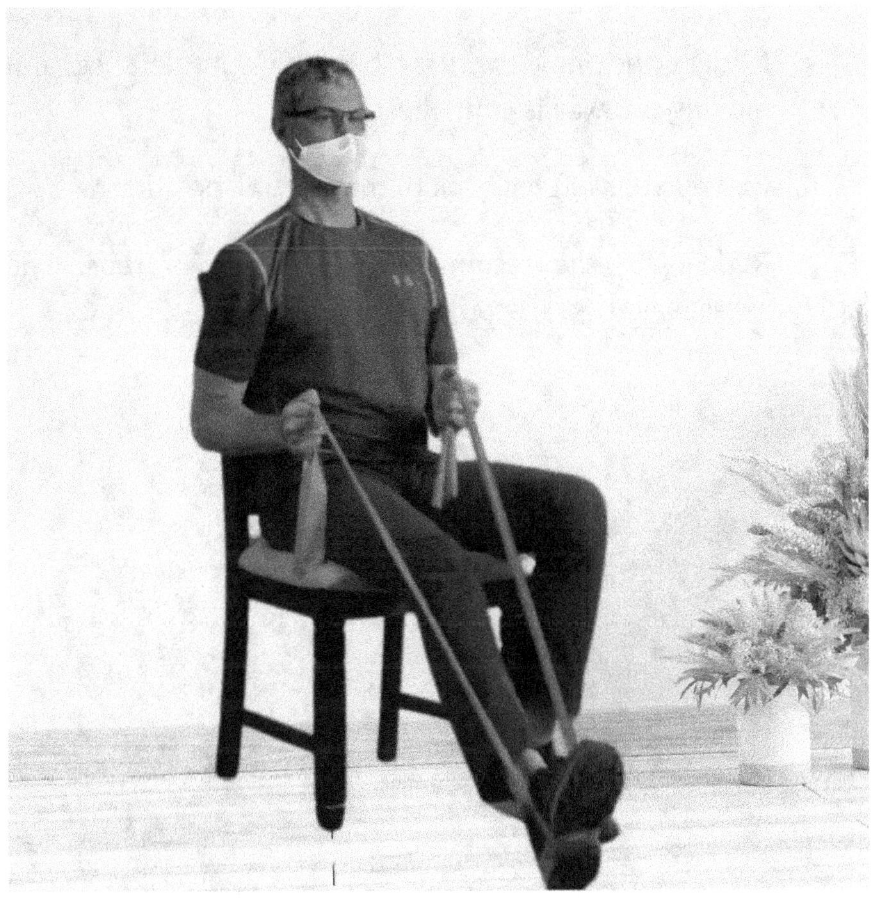

Here are the steps to do this exercise with a resistance band:

1. Sit upright in your chair with your shoulders down and back.

2. Hold both ends of the resistance band in your hands.

3. Place the band in the middle of the sole on your left foot.

4. Extend your left leg in front of you while firmly planting your right foot on the ground.

5. Initiate the movement by bending your left leg and moving it towards your chest.

6. Extend your left leg back to the starting position.

7. Repeat for the recommended amount of reps. The average is 10–15 repetitions per side.

Calf Press

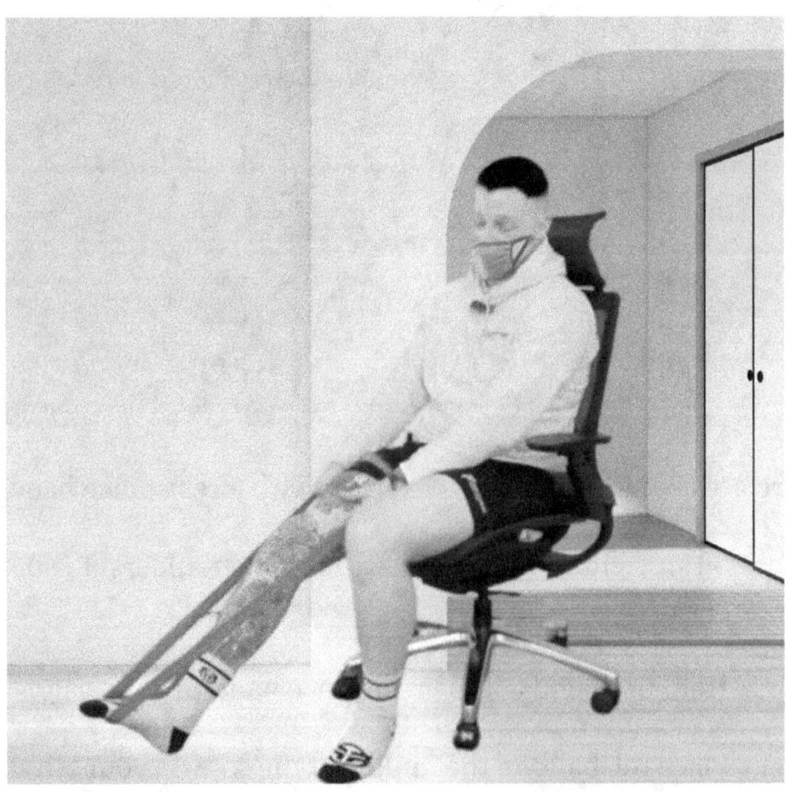

Here are the steps to do this exercise with a resistance band:

1. Sit upright in your chair with your shoulders down and back.

2. Hold both ends of the resistance band in your hands.

3. Place the band in the middle of the sole on your left foot.

4. Extend your left leg in front of you while firmly planting your right foot on the ground.

5. Initiate the movement by flexing your left foot forward toward the ground from the ankle.

6. Flex your toes upwards toward the ceiling.

7. Repeat for the recommended amount of reps. The average is 10–15 repetitions per side.

Leg Extension

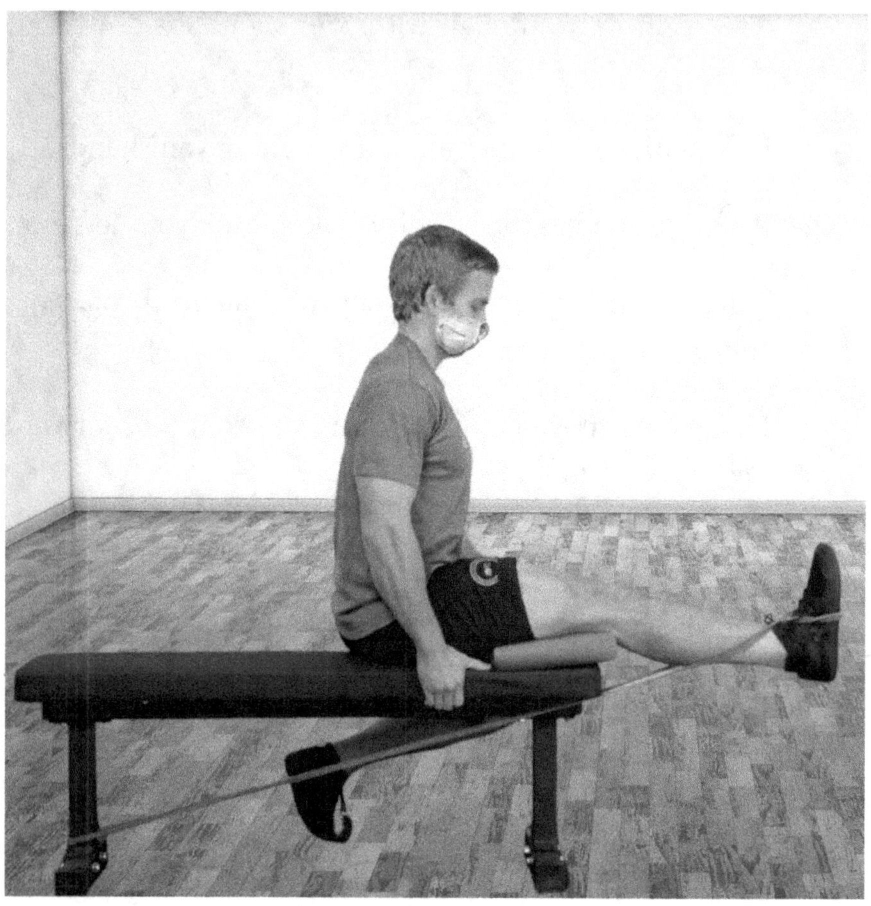

Here are the steps to do this exercise with a resistance band:

1. Sit upright in your chair with your shoulders down and back.

2. Place one end of the resistance band on the left back leg of your chair and the other end on your left ankle.

3. Keep both feet underneath your knees, but create tension on the band so it is slightly taut against your ankle.

4. Shift your weight to your right foot and lift your right leg from the floor.

5. Extend your left knee until it straightens out in front of you.

6. Return to the starting position.

7. Repeat for the recommended amount of reps. The average is 8–12 repetitions per side.

Sitting Leg Curl

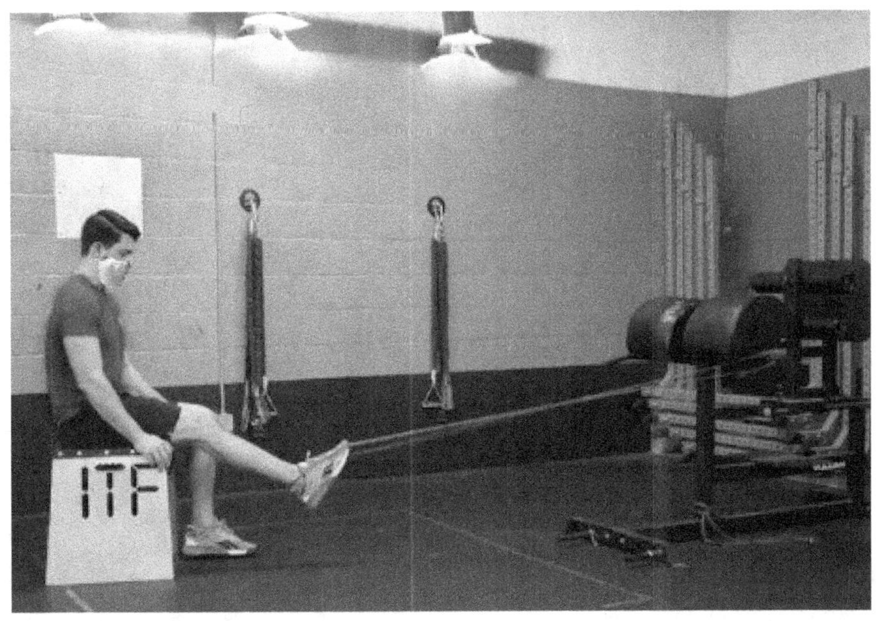

Here are the steps to do this exercise with a resistance band:

1. Anchor the resistance band at a point close to the floor.

2. Sit in a chair and loop the band around your right ankle.

3. Move away from the anchor to create tension in the band.

4. Bend your right knee, bringing your heel towards your glutes as far as comfortable.

5. Return your leg to the starting position.

6. Repeat for the recommended amount of reps. The average is 10–15 repetitions per side.

Clamshells

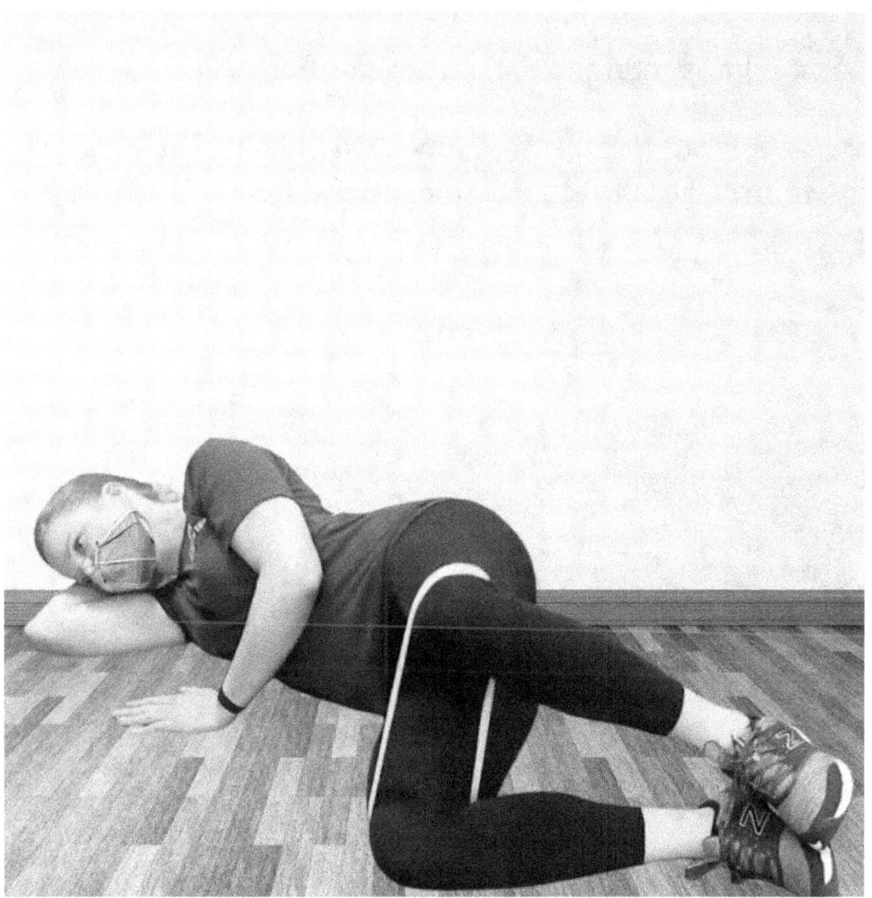

Here are the steps to do this exercise with a resistance band:

1. Loop a band around your legs just above your knees.

2. Sit in a chair or lie on the floor on your side, with one leg on top of the other and your knees slightly bent.

3. Keep your feet together and pull your knees away from each other while squeezing your glutes for 2–3 seconds.

4. Slowly return to the starting position.

5. Repeat for the recommended amount of reps. The average is 10–12 repetitions per side.

Banded Lateral Walks

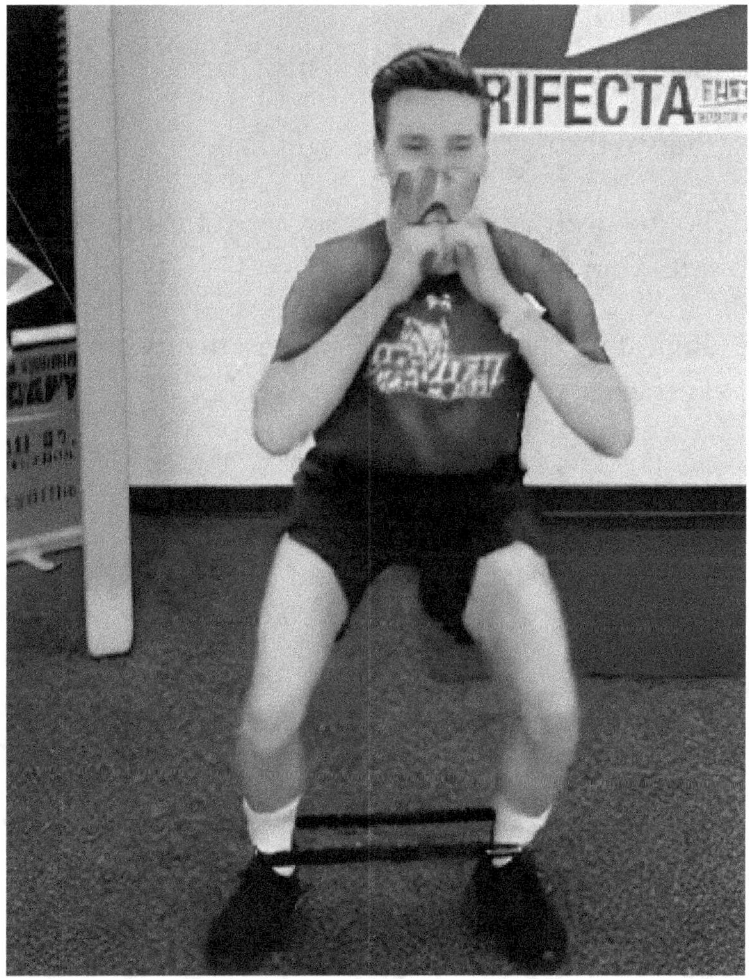

Here are the steps to do this exercise with a resistance band:

1. Begin by standing up tall with your shoulders back and down. Engage your core.

2. Your feet should be hip-width apart. Place a band around the top of your ankles.

3. Bend slightly at your knees into a partial squat.

4. Step to the right with your right foot.

5. Follow with your left foot so you return to the middle with your feet hip-width apart.

6. Repeat for the recommended reps, then swap sides. The average is 10–15 repetitions per side.

Glute Bridge

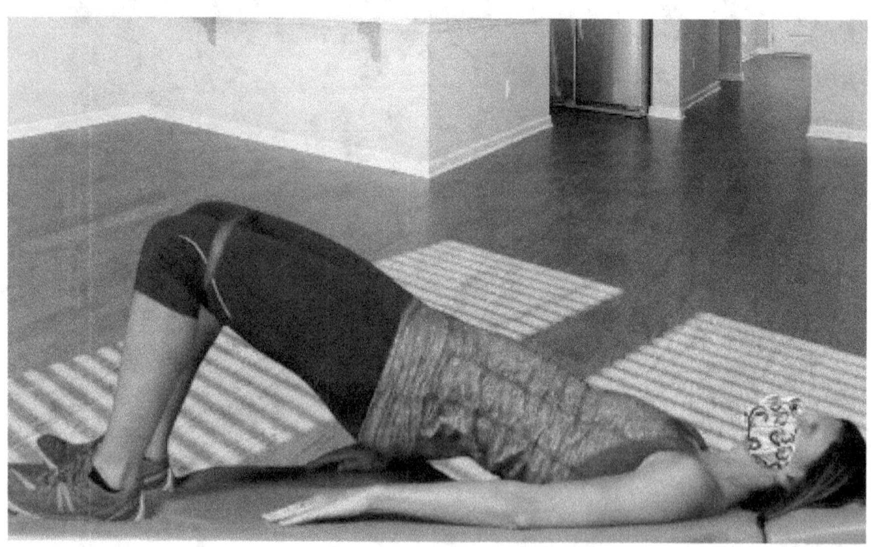

Here are the steps to do this exercise with resistance band:

1. Begin by lying flat on your back.

2. Place the resistance band above your knees.

3. Position your feet flat on the floor with your knees at a 90° angle, and place your heels just outside your glutes.

4. Lift your hips by contracting your glutes.

5. As you raise them, apply outward pressure from your knees against the band.

6. Repeat for the recommended amount of reps. The average is 15–20 repetitions.

Full Body Exercises

Pallof Press

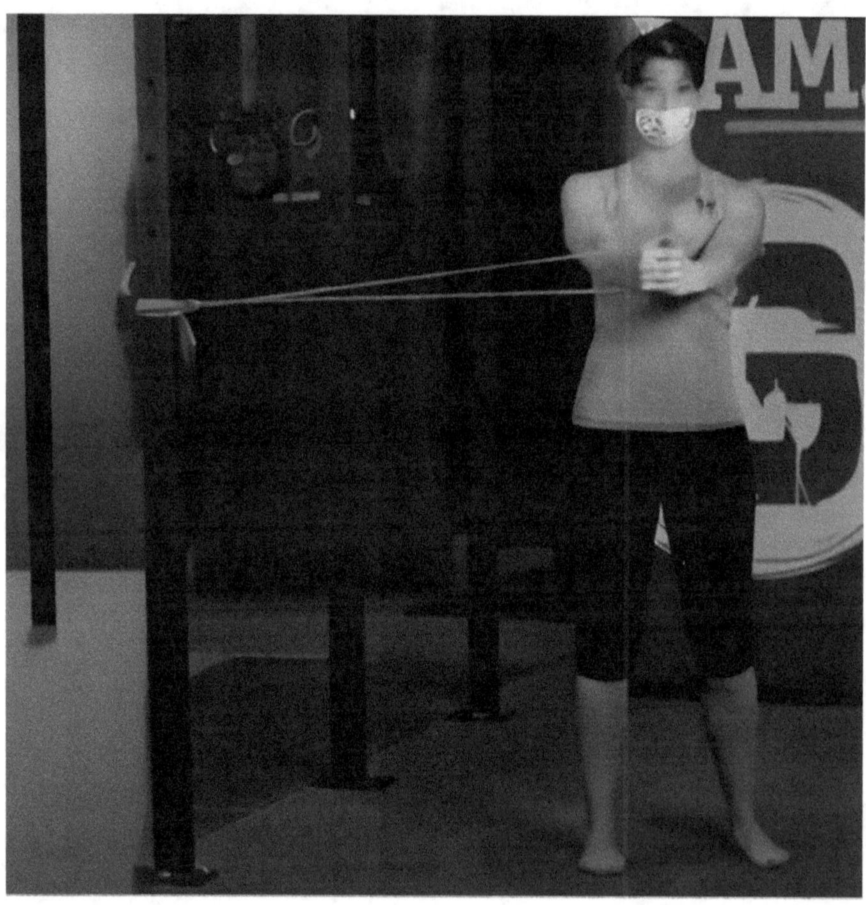

Here are the steps to do this exercise with resistance band:

1. Sit tall in a chair next to a door or anchor point where you will anchor your resistance band.

2. Anchor your band so that it is chest height.

3. Hold the resistance band in both hands and position yourself so there is tension on the band, slightly pulling you toward the anchor point.

4. Place your knees shoulder-width apart and hold the handle with your hands in front of you.

5. Brace your core and slowly press your hands in front of you until they are straight.

6. Pause for a second and return them to your chest.

7. Repeat for the recommended amount of reps, and then swap sides. The average is 8–12 repetitions per side.

Woodchopper

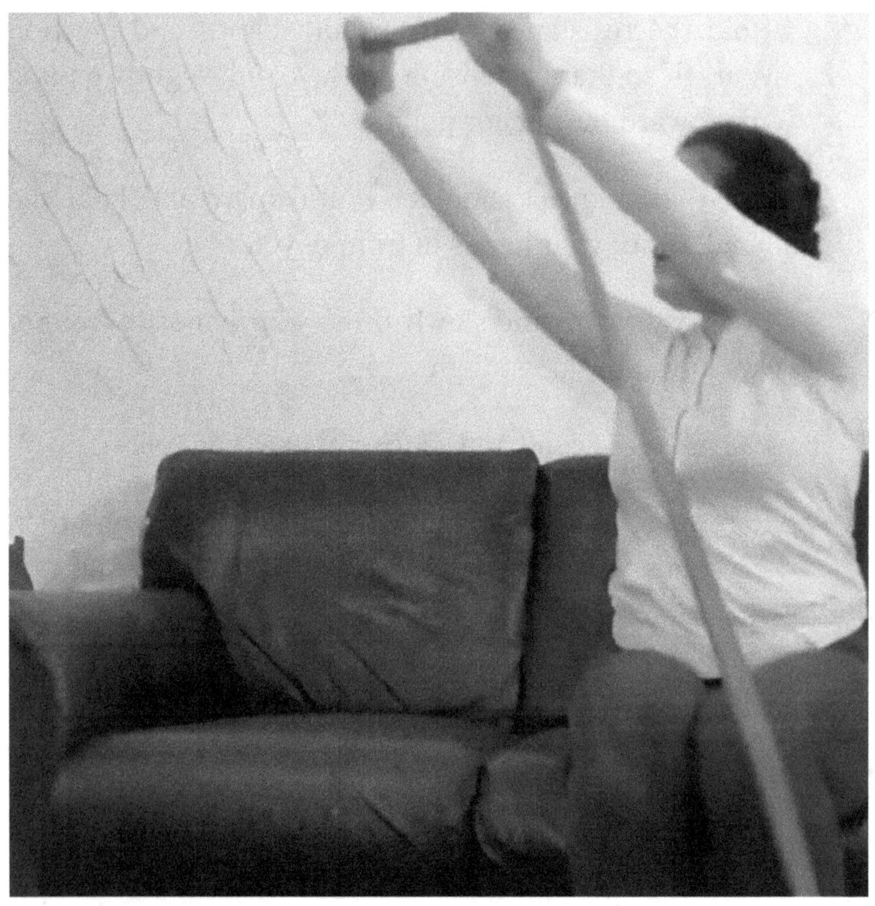

Here are the steps to do this exercise with resistance band:

1. Anchor the band close to the floor on a stable and secure object.

2. Adjust the chair to provide the required resistance at the starting position. Keep your chest up and core activated.

3. Stand with your feet shoulder-width apart, arms straight, and hanging down towards your left foot.

4. Pull the band diagonally towards the right, extending it overhead in a chopping motion. Allow your hips to gently twist and your left foot to pivot.

5. Lower your arms back to the starting position.

6. Repeat for the recommended amount of reps, then swap sides. The average is 8–10 repetitions per side.

Anti-Rotation Band Walkout

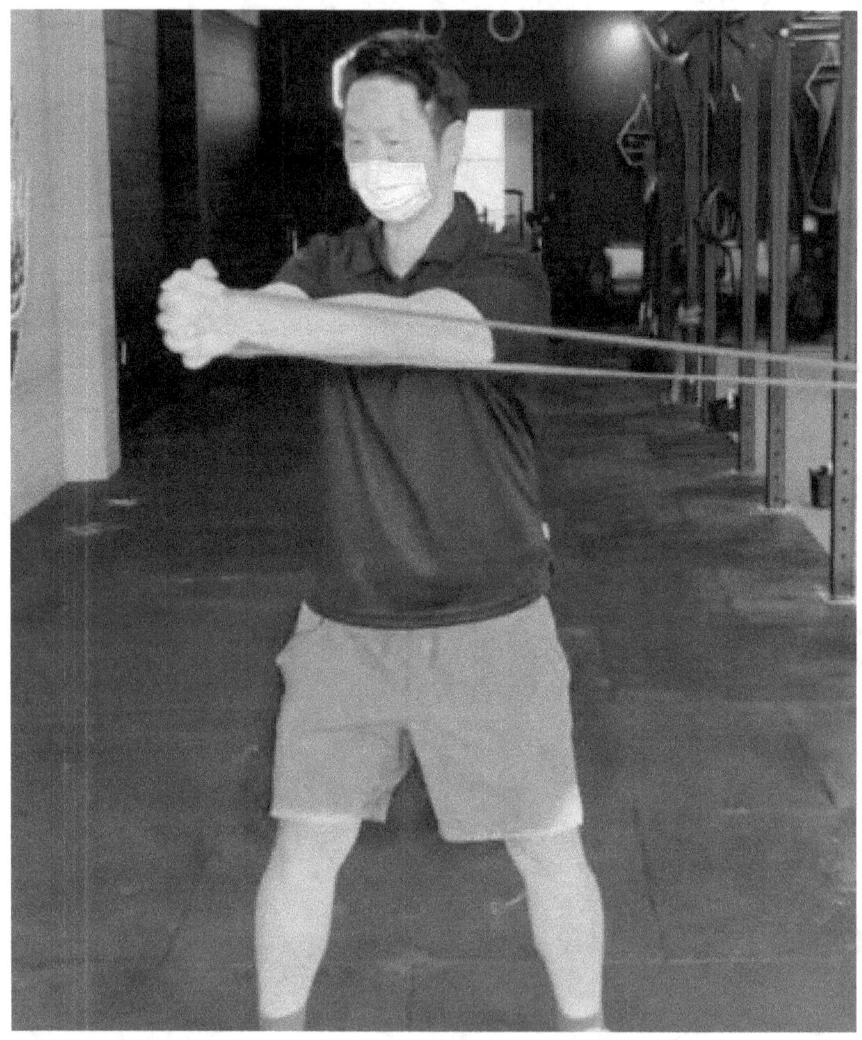

Here are the steps to do this exercise with resistance band:

1. Begin by anchoring your resistance band to a chest-high door or pillar.

2. Keep the band to the outside of your body and hold onto the other end with both hands.

3. Move away from the anchor point to create tension in the band.

4. Bend your knees slightly, getting into a partial squat position.

5. Hold the band with both hands straight out in front of your chest.

6. Step sideways away from the band until it is too tense to go any further.

7. Slowly move back toward the anchor point to return to the starting position.

8. Repeat for the recommended amount of reps, and then swap sides. The average is 6–8 repetitions per side.

Russian Twist

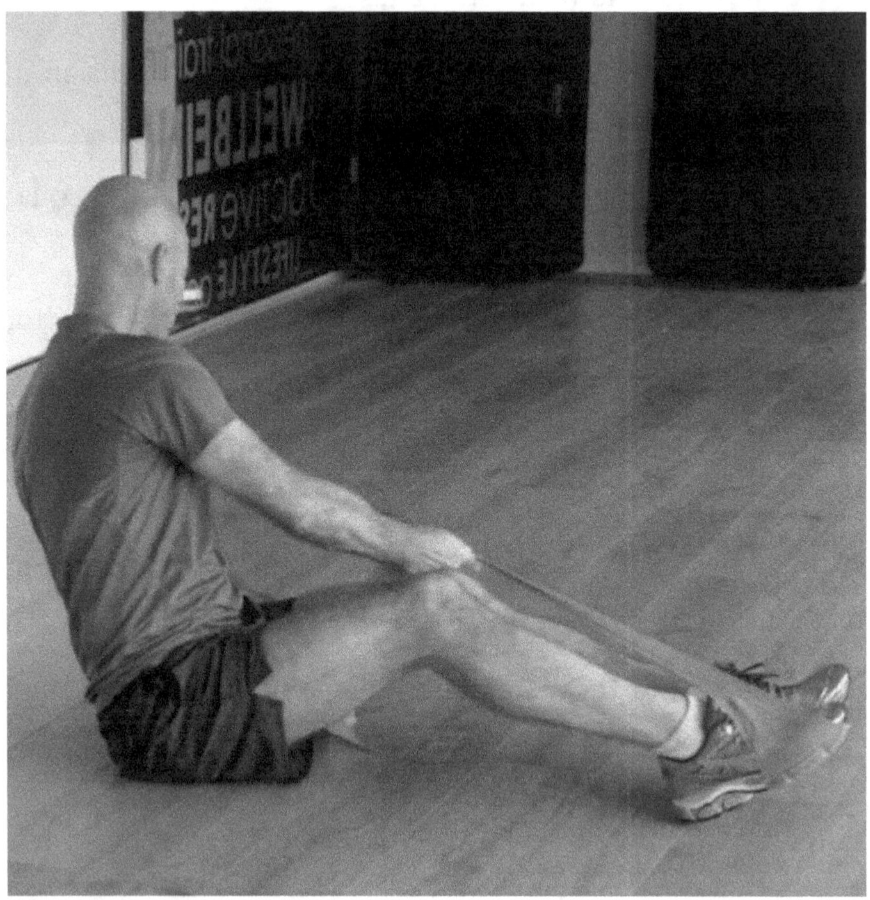

Here are the steps to do this exercise with a resistance band:

1. Begin by sitting tall in your chair or sitting on the floor with your legs out in front of you, knees slightly bent.

2. Loop the center of the resistance band around the soles of your feet and hold the other end with both hands.

3. Gently lean back at a 45° angle, keeping your arms straight in front of you and aligned with your chest.

4. While keeping the back of your heels on the floor, rotate from your hips towards your right side, bringing your hands to just outside your right hip.

5. Rotate back to the center and then to the left side. This completes one repetition.

6. Repeat the twisting motion for the recommended amount of reps. The average is 10–12 repetitions.

Banded Bicycle Crunch

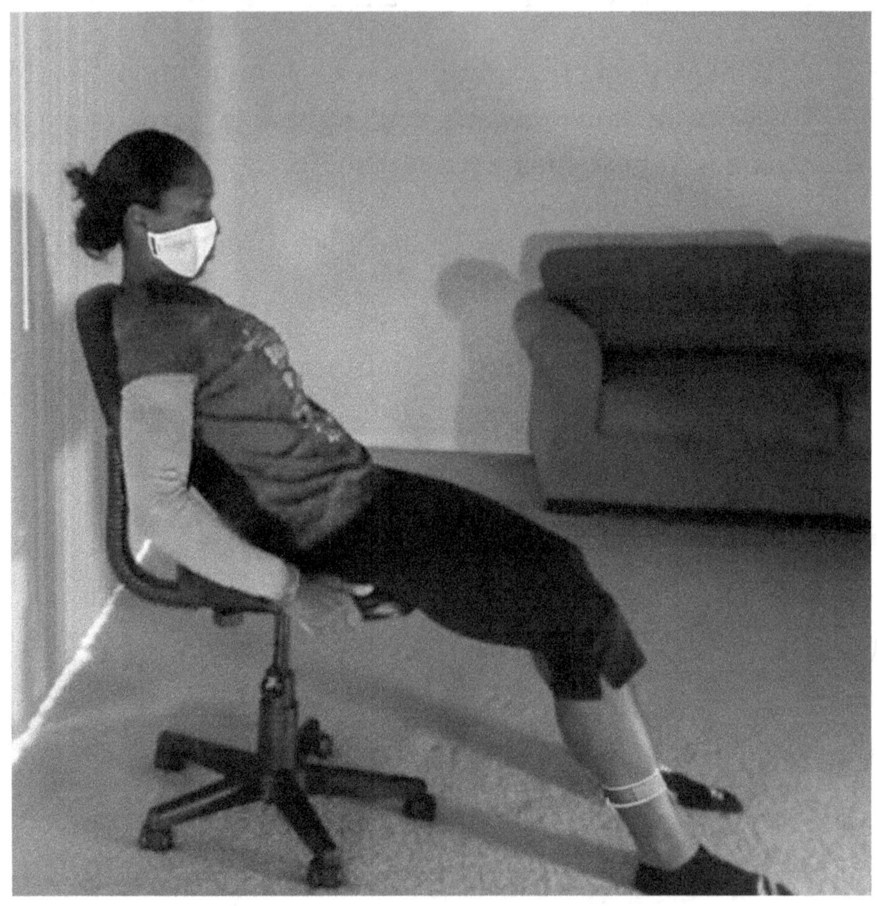

Here are the steps to do this exercise with resistance band:

1. Begin by sitting up tall in your chair.

2. Loop a short resistance band around your feet.

3. Place your hands behind your butt and lean back at a 45-degree angle.

4. Extend your right foot out while pulling your left knee towards your chest.

5. Swap sides, extending your left foot out and pulling your right knee towards your chest.

6. Repeat this pedaling motion for the recommended amount of reps. The average is 10–12 repetitions per side.

Banded Bird Dog

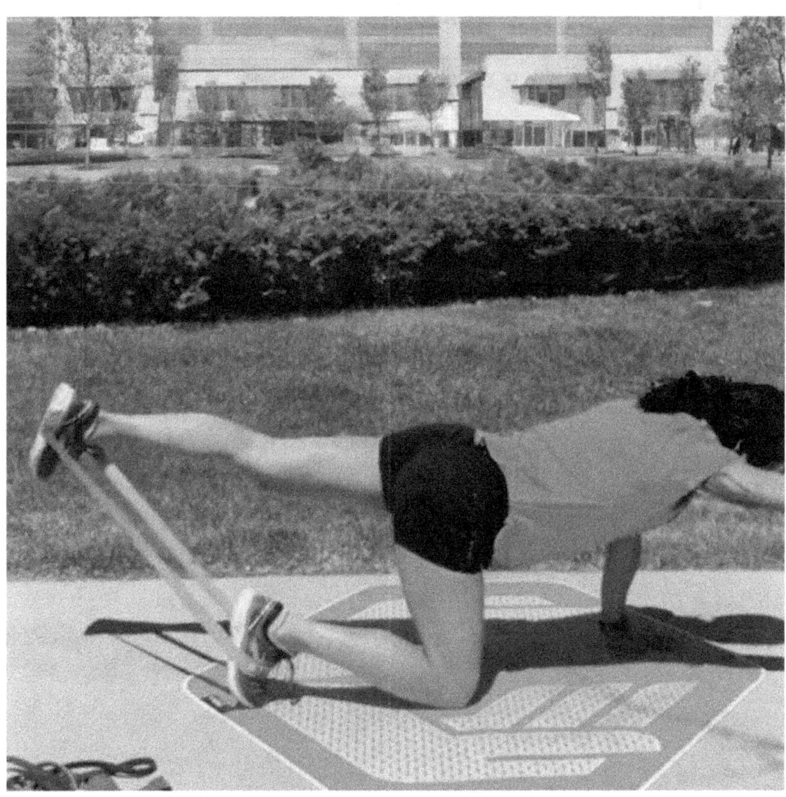

Here are the steps to do this exercise with a resistance band:

1. Begin on all fours with your knees underneath your hips and your palms underneath your shoulders. Keep your back straight and engage your midline.

2. Place a resistance band on both feet at the arches.

3. Extend your left leg straight behind you, barely touching your left toe to the floor.

4. Pull your left leg back, bringing your knee towards the floor.

5. Repeat the same movement with your right leg.

6. Continue alternating between the left and right legs for the recommended reps. The average is 8–12 repetitions per side.

Penguin Crunch

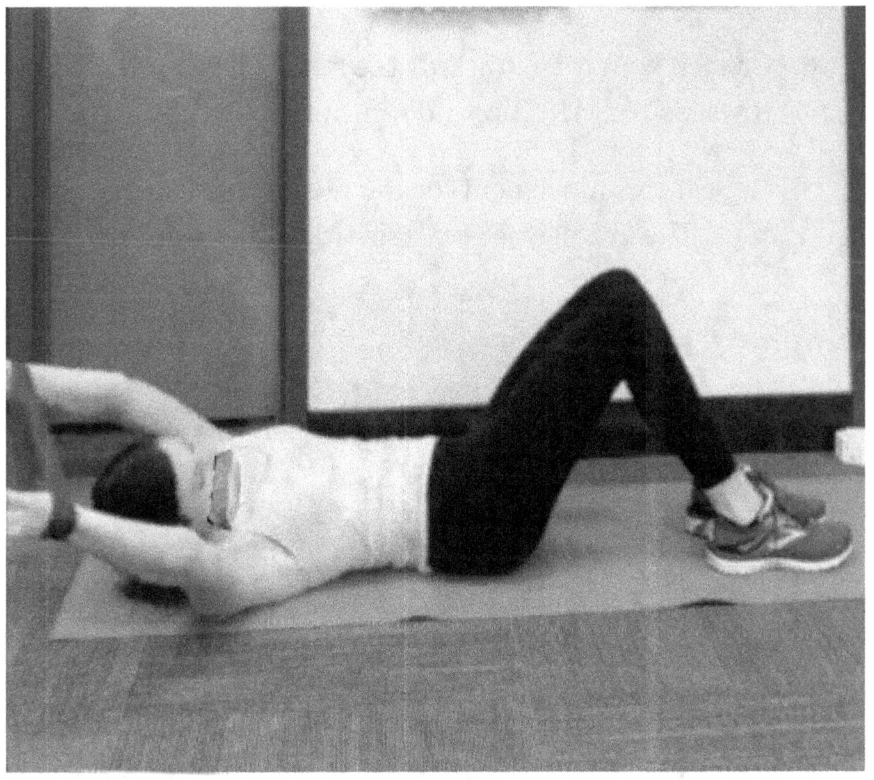

Here are the steps to do this exercise with a resistance band:

1. Start by lying on your back with the resistance band in each hand, keeping it taut.

2. Bend your knees and keep your feet flat on the floor.

3. Slowly raise your shoulders off the ground, maintaining tension in the band.

4. Extend your arms overhead.

5. Crunch your torso towards the right, bring your right elbow towards your right hip, and return to the center.

6. Crunch your torso towards the left, bring your left elbow towards your left hip, and return to the center.

7. Repeat this movement for the recommended amount of reps. The average is 8–12 repetitions per side.

Donkey Kick

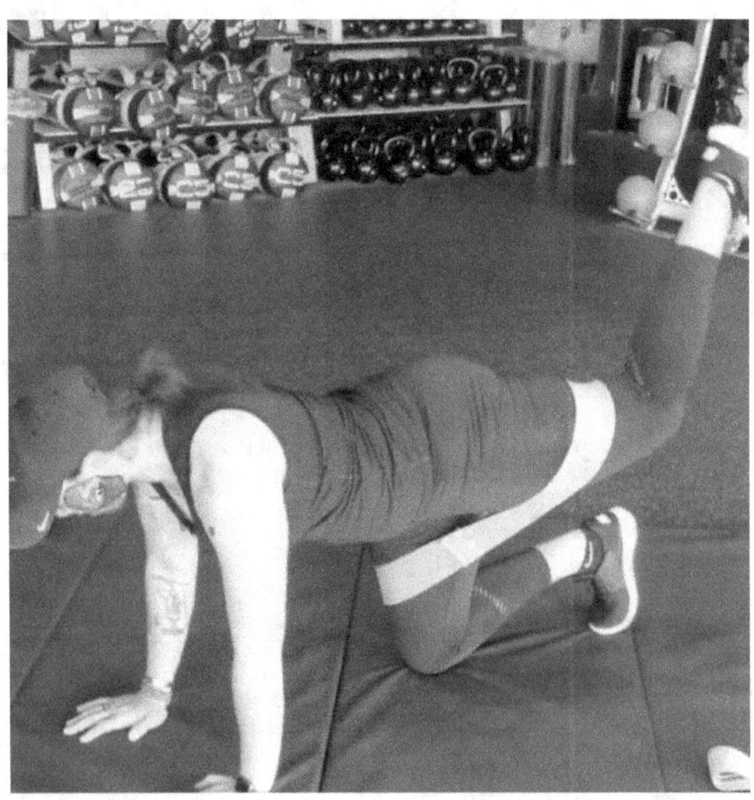

Here are the steps to do this exercise with a resistance band:

1. Start on all fours with your knees under your hips and your palms under your shoulders, maintaining a straight back and engaged core.

2. Place the resistance band around your thighs, just above the knee.

3. Lift your right leg off the floor, extending it backward and kicking your foot toward the ceiling.

4. Keep your leg in line with your hip, engaging your glutes and maintaining tension in the band.

5. Return your right leg to the starting position.

6. Swap legs and repeat the same movement with your left leg.

7. Continue alternating legs for the recommended amount of reps. The average is 8–12 repetitions per side.

CHAPTER 4: 28-DAYS CHALLENGE

Join our 28-day Resistance Band Challenge to enhance your strength and flexibility.

This plan is designed for seniors and includes a variety of exercises using resistance bands. Each day focuses on different areas of the body - upper body, lower body, and full-body workouts. Whether you are a beginner or already active, this plan is suitable for all fitness levels. Experience gradual improvements in your strength and overall well-being.

Get ready to engage in new exercises, boost your energy levels, and enjoy the Resistance Band Challenge for the upcoming month!

Week 1

Day 1

Warm Up Exercise:

Marching - 5 mins

Resistance Band Exercises:

Band Pull Aparts - 3 sets of 12 reps

Lateral Raise - 3 sets of 12 reps

Seated Row - 3 sets of 12 reps

Banded Squat #1 - 3 sets of 12 reps

Pallof Press - 3 sets of 10 reps/side

Cool Down Exercise:

Cat/Cow Stretch - 3 sets of 15 secs

Day 2

Warm Up Exercise:

Walking Jacks - 5 mins

Resistance Band Exercises:

Bent Over Row - 3 sets of 12 reps

Overhead Press - 3 sets of 10 reps

Banded Squat #2 - 3 sets of 12 reps

Woodchopper - 3 sets of 12 reps/side

Russian Twist - 3 sets of 15 reps/side

Cool Down Exercise:

Forward Bend - 3 sets of 15 secs

Day 3

Warm Up Exercise:

Knees to Elbow Marching - 5 mins

Resistance Band Exercises:

Overhead Triceps Extension - 3 sets of 12 reps

Deadlift - 3 sets of 12 reps

Kickstand Single-Leg-Romanian Deadlift - 3 sets of 12 reps/side

Anti-Rotation Band Walkout - 3 sets of 8 reps/side

Seated Hip Lateral Rotation Stretch - 3 sets of 15 secs

Cool Down Exercise:

Hamstring Stretch - 3 sets of 15 secs

Day 4

Warm Up Exercise:

Shadow Boxing - 5 mins

Resistance Band Exercises:

Biceps Curl - 3 sets of 15 reps

Upright Row - 3 sets of 12 reps

Standing Adduction - 3 sets of 15 reps/side

Russian Twist - 3 sets of 15 reps/side

Seated Hip Flexion Stretch - 3 sets of 15 secs

Cool Down Exercise:

Quadruped Stretch - 3 sets of 15 secs

Day 5

Warm Up Exercise:

Lateral Side Steps - 5 mins

Resistance Band Exercises:

Seated Row - 3 sets of 12 reps

Cuff Pivot - 3 sets of 10 reps/side

Chest Press - 3 sets of 12 reps

Clamshells - 3 sets of 15 reps/side

Abductor Stretch - 3 sets of 15 secs

Cool Down Exercise:

Calf Stretch - 3 sets of 15 secs

Day 6

Warm Up Exercise:

Head Rolls - 3 mins

Resistance Band Exercises:

Banded Front Raise - 3 sets of 12 reps

Scapular Retraction - 3 sets of 12 reps

Overhead Pull Apart - 3 sets of 12 reps

Leg Press - 3 sets of 15 reps

Banded Lateral Walks - 3 sets of 15 reps/side

Cool Down Exercise:

Lumbar Side Stretch - 3 sets of 15 secs

Day 7

Warm Up Exercise:

Neck Rotations - 3 mins

Resistance Band Exercises:

Cuff Pivot - 3 sets of 10 reps/side

Chest Press - 3 sets of 12 reps

Seated Hip Lateral Rotation Stretch - 3 sets of 15 secs

Russian Twist - 3 sets of 15 reps/side

Forward Bend - 3 sets of 15 secs

Cool Down Exercise:

Quadruped Stretch - 3 sets of 15 secs

Week 2

Day 8

Warm Up Exercise:

Lateral Flexion - 3 mins

Resistance Band Exercises:

Overhead Press - 3 sets of 10 reps

Cuff Pivot - 3 sets of 10 reps/side

Overhead Triceps Extension - 3 sets of 12 reps

Standing Adduction - 3 sets of 15 reps/side

Calf Stretch - 3 sets of 15 secs

Cool Down Exercise:

Hamstring Stretch - 3 sets of 15 secs

Day 9

Warm Up Exercise:

Wrist Rotation - 3 mins

Resistance Band Exercises:

Biceps Curl - 3 sets of 15 reps

Cuff Pivot - 3 sets of 10 reps/side

Scapular Retraction - 3 sets of 12 reps

Banded Squat #2 - 3 sets of 12 reps

Anti-Rotation Band Walkout - 3 sets of 8 reps/side

Cool Down Exercise:

Seated Hip Lateral Rotation Stretch - 3 sets of 15 secs

Day 10

Warm Up Exercise:

Forearm Circles - 3 mins

Resistance Band Exercises:

Upright Row - 3 sets of 12 reps

Overhead Pull Apart - 3 sets of 12 reps

Banded Front Raise - 3 sets of 12 reps

Pallof Press - 3 sets of 10 reps/side

Hamstring Stretch - 3 sets of 15 secs

Cool Down Exercise:

Quadruped Stretch - 3 sets of 15 secs

Day 11

Warm Up Exercise:

Arm Circles - 3 mins

Resistance Band Exercises:

Cuff Pivot - 3 sets of 10 reps/side

Chest Press - 3 sets of 12 reps

Seated Hip Flexion Stretch - 3 sets of 15 secs

Banded Squat #1 - 3 sets of 12 reps

Seated Hip Lateral Rotation Stretch - 3 sets of 15 secs

Cool Down Exercise:

Forward Bend - 3 sets of 15 secs

Day 12

Warm Up Exercise:

Marching - 5 mins

Resistance Band Exercises:

Overhead Triceps Extension - 3 sets of 12 reps

Lateral Raise - 3 sets of 12 reps

Seated Row - 3 sets of 12 reps

Banded Squat #1 - 3 sets of 12 reps

Pallof Press - 3 sets of 10 reps/side

Cool Down Exercise:

Cat/Cow Stretch - 3 sets of 15 secs

Day 13

Warm Up Exercise:

Walking Jacks - 5 mins

Resistance Band Exercises:

Bent Over Row - 3 sets of 12 reps

Overhead Press - 3 sets of 10 reps

Banded Squat #2 - 3 sets of 12 reps

Woodchopper - 3 sets of 12 reps/side

Russian Twist - 3 sets of 15 reps/side

Cool Down Exercise:

Forward Bend - 3 sets of 15 secs

Day 14

Warm Up Exercise:

Knees to Elbow Marching - 5 mins

Resistance Band Exercises:

Overhead Triceps Extension - 3 sets of 12 reps

Deadlift - 3 sets of 12 reps

Kickstand Single-Leg-Romanian Deadlift - 3 sets of 12 reps/side

Anti-Rotation Band Walkout - 3 sets of 8 reps/side

Seated Hip Lateral Rotation Stretch - 3 sets of 15 secs

Cool Down Exercise:

Hamstring Stretch - 3 sets of 15 secs

Week 3

Day 15

Warm Up Exercise:

Shadow Boxing - 5 mins

Resistance Band Exercises:

Biceps Curl - 3 sets of 15 reps

Upright Row - 3 sets of 12 reps

Standing Adduction - 3 sets of 15 reps/side

Russian Twist - 3 sets of 15 reps/side

Seated Hip Flexion Stretch - 3 sets of 15 secs

Cool Down Exercise:

Quadruped Stretch - 3 sets of 15 secs

Day 16

Warm Up Exercise:

Lateral Side Steps - 5 mins

Resistance Band Exercises:

Seated Row - 3 sets of 12 reps

Cuff Pivot - 3 sets of 10 reps/side

Chest Press - 3 sets of 12 reps

Clamshells - 3 sets of 15 reps/side

Abductor Stretch - 3 sets of 15 secs

Cool Down Exercise:

Calf Stretch - 3 sets of 15 secs

Day 17

Warm Up Exercise:

Head Rolls - 3 mins

Resistance Band Exercises:

Banded Front Raise - 3 sets of 12 reps

Scapular Retraction - 3 sets of 12 reps

Overhead Pull Apart - 3 sets of 12 reps

Leg Press - 3 sets of 15 reps

Banded Lateral Walks - 3 sets of 15 reps/side

Cool Down Exercise:

Lumbar Side Stretch - 3 sets of 15 secs

Day 18

Warm Up Exercise:

Neck Rotations - 3 mins

Resistance Band Exercises:

Cuff Pivot - 3 sets of 10 reps/side

Chest Press - 3 sets of 12 reps

Seated Hip Lateral Rotation Stretch - 3 sets of 15 secs

Russian Twist - 3 sets of 15 reps/side

Forward Bend - 3 sets of 15 secs

Cool Down Exercise:

Quadruped Stretch - 3 sets of 15 secs

Day 19

Warm Up Exercise:

Neck Lateral Flexion - 3 mins

Resistance Band Exercises:

Overhead Press - 3 sets of 10 reps

Cuff Pivot - 3 sets of 10 reps/side

Overhead Triceps Extension - 3 sets of 12 reps

Standing Adduction - 3 sets of 15 reps/side

Calf Stretch - 3 sets of 15 secs

Cool Down Exercise:

Hamstring Stretch - 3 sets of 15 secs

Day 20

Warm Up Exercise:

Wrist Rotation - 3 mins

Resistance Band Exercises:

Biceps Curl - 3 sets of 15 reps

Cuff Pivot - 3 sets of 10 reps/side

Scapular Retraction - 3 sets of 12 reps

Banded Squat #2 - 3 sets of 12 reps

Anti-Rotation Band Walkout - 3 sets of 8 reps/side

Cool Down Exercise:

Seated Hip Lateral Rotation Stretch - 3 sets of 15 secs

Day 21

Warm Up Exercise:

Forearm Circles - 3 mins

Resistance Band Exercises:

Upright Row - 3 sets of 12 reps

Overhead Pull Apart - 3 sets of 12 reps

Banded Front Raise - 3 sets of 12 reps

Pallof Press - 3 sets of 10 reps/side

Hamstring Stretch - 3 sets of 15 secs

Cool Down Exercise:

Quadruped Stretch - 3 sets of 15 secs

Week 4

Day 22

Warm Up Exercise:

Arm Circles - 3 mins

Resistance Band Exercises:

Cuff Pivot - 3 sets of 10 reps/side

Chest Press - 3 sets of 12 reps

Seated Hip Flexion Stretch - 3 sets of 15 secs

Banded Squat #1 - 3 sets of 12 reps

Seated Hip Lateral Rotation Stretch - 3 sets of 15 secs

Cool Down Exercise:

Forward Bend - 3 sets of 15 secs

Day 23

Warm Up Exercise:

Marching - 5 mins

Resistance Band Exercises:

Overhead Triceps Extension - 3 sets of 12 reps

Lateral Raise - 3 sets of 12 reps

Seated Row - 3 sets of 12 reps

Banded Squat #1 - 3 sets of 12 reps

Pallof Press - 3 sets of 10 reps/side

Cool Down Exercise:

Cat/Cow Stretch - 3 sets of 15 secs

Day 24

Warm Up Exercise:

Walking Jacks - 5 mins

Resistance Band Exercises:

Bent Over Row - 3 sets of 12 reps

Overhead Press - 3 sets of 10 reps

Banded Squat #2 - 3 sets of 12 reps

Woodchopper - 3 sets of 12 reps/side

Russian Twist - 3 sets of 15 reps/side

Cool Down Exercise:

Forward Bend - 3 sets of 15 secs

Day 25

Warm Up Exercise:

Knees to Elbow Marching - 5 mins

Resistance Band Exercises:

Overhead Triceps Extension - 3 sets of 12 reps

Deadlift - 3 sets of 12 reps

Kickstand Single-Leg-Romanian Deadlift - 3 sets of 12 reps/side

Anti-Rotation Band Walkout - 3 sets of 8 reps/side

Seated Hip Lateral Rotation Stretch - 3 sets of 15 secs

Cool Down Exercise:

Hamstring Stretch - 3 sets of 15 secs

Day 26

Warm Up Exercise:

Shadow Boxing - 5 mins

Resistance Band Exercises:

Biceps Curl - 3 sets of 15 reps

Upright Row - 3 sets of 12 reps

Standing Adduction - 3 sets of 15 reps/side

Russian Twist - 3 sets of 15 reps/side

Seated Hip Flexion Stretch - 3 sets of 15 secs

Cool Down Exercise:

Quadruped Stretch - 3 sets of 15 secs

Day 27

Warm Up Exercise:

Lateral Side Steps - 5 mins

Resistance Band Exercises:

Seated Row - 3 sets of 12 reps

Cuff Pivot - 3 sets of 10 reps/side

Chest Press - 3 sets of 12 reps

Clamshells - 3 sets of 15 reps/side

Abductor Stretch - 3 sets of 15 secs

Cool Down Exercise:

Calf Stretch - 3 sets of 15 secs

Day 28

Warm Up Exercise:

Head Rolls - 3 mins

Resistance Band Exercises:

Banded Front Raise - 3 sets of 12 reps

Scapular Retraction - 3 sets of 12 reps

Overhead Pull Apart - 3 sets of 12 reps

Leg Press - 3 sets of 15 reps

Banded Lateral Walks - 3 sets of 15 reps/side

Cool Down Exercise:

Lumbar Side Stretch - 3 sets of 15 secs

CONCLUSION

I want to give you a big round of applause. Starting a journey towards better health and vitality from scratch takes work. Congratulations on taking control of your health and embracing exercise – a crucial step towards a new quality of life and a positive outlook.

With determination and commitment, you'll show that age is not a barrier to achieving strength, flexibility, and well-being.

Throughout this book, we've explored the many benefits of resistance band exercises, showing that you have the power to transform your life through simple yet effective workouts. By adding these exercises to your daily routines, you're improving your physical health and boosting your mental and emotional well-being.

Remember, every stretch, every rep, and every time you push beyond your comfort zone is a sign of your resilience and determination. It's making you healthier and giving you the vitality and longevity you deserve.

The same principles apply to your nutrition, sleep, and stress management. Taking care of these aspects creates holistic wellness, and as you dive deeper into your healthy lifestyle, these pieces will align and fall into place together.

Your commitment to your well-being is truly inspiring. It's never too late to start, and with each workout and every healthy meal, you're rewriting the narrative of aging.

As you continue on this path, may you find strength in every challenge, joy in every achievement, and a renewed sense of vitality that empowers you to live life to the fullest.

Keep moving, and keep believing in the incredible potential within you. The best is yet to come!

www.ingramcontent.com/pod-product-compliance
Lightning Source LLC
Chambersburg PA
CBHW070759260726
48660CB00005B/1693